Sick Building Syndrome
and the Problem of Uncertainty

Michelle Murphy

Sick Building Syndrome and the Problem of Uncertainty

Environmental Politics, Technoscience, and Women Workers

DUKE UNIVERSITY PRESS Durham and London 2006

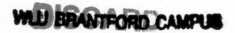

Designed by C. H. Westmoreland
Typeset in Scala and Arial
by Keystone Typesetting, Inc.
Diesel display font by Eduardo Recife
(www.misprintedtype.com)
Library of Congress Cataloging-in-
Publication Data appear on the last printed
page of this book.

Duke University Press gratefully

acknowledges the support of the Graham

Foundation for Advanced Studies in the Fine Arts,

which provided funds for the production and

distribution of this book.

To Matt

Contents

Acknowledgments   ix

Introduction   1

[1]   Man in a Box: Building-Machines and
the Science of Comfort   19

[2]   Building Ladies into the Office Machine   35

[3]   Feminism, Surveys, and Toxic Details   57

[4]   Indoor Pollution at the Encounter of Toxicology
and Popular Epidemiology   81

[5]   Uncertainty, Race, and Activism at the EPA   111

[6]   Building Ecologies, Tobacco, and the Politics
of Multiplicity   131

[7]   How to Build Yourself a Body in a Safe Space   151

Epilogue   179

Notes   181

Bibliography   213

Index   241

Acknowledgments

First a seminar paper, then a dissertation, and now finally a book, *Sick Building Syndrome and the Problem of Uncertainty* has been brewing for a decade. It is thus not surprising that I have accrued many debts of gratitude along the way. The faculty and graduate students at the Department of History of Science at Harvard University provided a provoking environment in which to conceptualize, research, and write about twentieth-century science and the history of how things come to matter. In particular, I would like to thank Allan Brandt, Peter Galison, Barbara Rosenkrantz, Katherine Park, Everett Mendelsohn, Carl Pearson, Wendy Lynch, Conevery Bolton Valencius, Alex Cooper, Nick Weiss, Nick King, and Lisa Herschbach. From my time at Cambridge to the present, Evelynn Hammonds has been both an intellectual mentor and a guide in the struggle to remain politicized and grounded as an academic. During a postdoctoral fellowship at the Max Planck Institute for the History of Science, I met many excellent scholars to whom I am deeply grateful for helping me to sharpen this work, including Sabine Holer, Abigail Lustig, Jens Lachmund, Robert Proctor, and especially Lorraine Daston, who set a standard of scholarship that is truly inspirational. Gregg Mitman has profoundly enriched my understanding of the history of environmental health, and I am grateful for his example of how to be both an excellent scholar and a good person. I would like also to thank the colleagues and friends who have read various versions of chapters over the years or have extended a patient ear, in particular Joe Dumit, Mike Fortun, Kim Fortun, Luciana Parisi, Michael Fitzhenry, Kristen Bucholz, Anna Greenspan, Adele Clarke, Nelly Oodshourn, Lisa Cartwright, Natalie Jeremijenko, Hannah Landecker, Chris Kelty, and Elspeth Brown. The participants in the Environmental Health in Global Perspective workshop at the University of Wisconsin, Madison, were instrumental in the refashioning of chapter 5, which I had wrestled over for many years. Also, thank you to my colleagues in the Department of History and the Women and Gender

Studies Institute at the University of Toronto for their support in helping me to finish this book.

During the researching, writing, and rewriting of this book, I was fortunate to receive a D. O. Robeson Graduate Scholarship for History at the University of Toronto; a Graduate Society Fellowship at Harvard University; a doctoral fellowship from the Social Sciences and Humanities Research Council of Canada; and an Eliot Dissertation Completion Grant from Harvard. I would like to thank the staff at the Schlesinger Archive, as well as Jeanne Stellman and 9to5 for granting me access to their collections there. I am deeply appreciative for the generous help extended to me by NFFE local 2050, particularly by William Hirzy. Thank you to the following people at the Environmental Protection Agency and elsewhere for granting me interviews and providing me with materials: Robert Axelrad, Kirby Biggs, Jeff Davidson, Claire Gilbert, Albert Donnay, Deborah Jaynes, James Repace, Cindy Richards, John Sprengler, Lance Wallace, and Susan Womble. Thank you to Reynolds Smith at Duke University Press for his editorial guidance.

Portions of chapter 3 were published previously by Taylor and Francis as "Toxicity in the Details: The History of the Women's Office Worker Movement and Occupational Health in the Late Capitalist Office" in *Labor History* 41, no. 2 (2000): 189–213; of chapter 5 by University of Chicago Press as "Uncertain Exposures and the Privilege of Imperception: Activist Scientists and Race at the U.S. Environmental Protection Agency" in *Osiris* 19 (2004): 266–82; and of chapter 7 by Johns Hopkins University Press as "The 'Elsewhere within Here' and Environmental Illness; or, How to Build Yourself a Body in a Safe Space" in *Configurations* 8, no. 1 (2000): 87–120. Thank you to these presses for their permission to republish this material.

Finally, I would like to thank my family for all their support, love, and patience, especially my parents Ted and Claudette Murphy, as well as Richard and Ellen Price. I am thankful to my two kids for turning out so wonderfully despite the fact that I wrote and rewrote this book bouncing them in one hand and typing with the other. Matt Price has read every line of every chapter at least once if not a dozen times. He is my most incisive critic, greatest advocate, and best friend. I dedicate this book to him.

Take a deep breath and hold it. Do you know that when you breathe in your lungs absorb billions upon billions of air molecules? Now breathe out.

Breathe in. Along with air, each lungful you inhale contains the detritus from our indoor environments: fibers, vapors, tiny airborne insects and their excrement, viruses, bacteria, and fungi. Breathe out.

Breathe in. Do you realize that chemical fumes from the objects around you escape into the air, are drawn into your lungs, dissolve across your alveoli membranes and into your blood? Breathe out.

Breathe in. The air you just inhaled has already passed through ducts encrusted with a grimy, gray, microbe-infested fuzz of debris, hair, dust, and fiber particles released by decaying building materials. Breathe out.—Classroom exercise from the Environmental Protection Agency designed to teach children about indoor air; paraphrase of Tchudi, "Lesson Plan on Indoor Air Quality" (1993)

Imagine an office building at the end of the twentieth century. One worker typing at a desk rubs an eye. Working in a nearby cubicle, a second blows a congested nose. Standing at the photocopier, a third passes a lozenge to a fourth. A fifth begins to feel dizzy as a coworker's perfume wafts by. A sixth, a seventh—a crowd of complaints begins to form.

Dispersed in far-flung corners of a building, these workers in the information economy at the end of the twentieth century may never have thought twice about their irritations. But sometimes they began talking to each other. Latent connections may already have been in place: maybe they were neighbors, or parishioners in the same church, or ate at the same table during lunch. Perhaps a first worker complained about an aspect of their work environment, and others chimed in—Me too, me three! Complaint comparison became a conversational buzz at breaks—

Me four, me five! Repetitions accumulated, and someone began asking questions, gathering in others: Do you feel unwell, too? Perhaps repetitions were recorded in a notebook, turned into signs that together gained new weight. Irritations absorbed into the crowd became symptoms, a collective pattern. Compelled by the din of complaints, other workers might also ask themselves questions about their own bodies. One can easily imagine prying open a ventilation grate and peering inside.

Suddenly a threshold was passed, and now many noticed that they felt unwell. A threshold was passed, and what yesterday had gone by without remark was today intolerable. The multitude continued to grow, giving work in the office building a new rhythm. Workers, mostly women, staged meetings, collected signatures, filed grievances, conducted informal surveys. What had been unconnected, diverse bodily occurrences cohered into an event. Individual symptoms joined the crowd of similarities and became linked in a chain of repetition: in the building . . . in the building . . . in the building. At other buildings, in other cities, strangely similar chains of events occurred. Though many miles apart, they heard news of each other through short newspaper articles or on TV. Workers in one building pointed to workers in other buildings. The crowd, linked by symptoms, declared an occupational health problem. A name circulated, under which all these differences coalesced: *sick building syndrome.*

Becoming Sick Building Syndrome

Before 1980, sick building syndrome did not exist. In order to become "sick," a certain kind of office building had to come into existence. In the 1970s, office buildings became architecturally "airtight" for the sake of energy efficiency, while internally they were arranged in "open" floor plans. Work inside was governed according to novel, cybernetics-inspired techniques of design and administration. New kinds of materials —plastics, solvents, adhesives, synthetic carpet, particle board, dry wall, acoustic tiles, and so on—made up the surfaces that in turn housed computers, printers, and fax machines that were mechanically kept cool and dry. Air-conditioned and carpeted, office buildings stood in striking contrast to the treacherous factories, pitiless sweatshops, and deadly mines of industrial work. Office buildings, constructed to house the vast extension of information work in booming postwar America, relied on a middle-class ambiance to delimit them as different from industrial workplaces, even if wages for many were comparable.

Sick building syndrome was a problem only possible in conditions of relative privilege and luxury that characterized Reagan-era America. It captured those minor health complaints only foregrounded when larger dangers receded. It expressed an expectation of comfort and safety as conditions of daily life for the beneficiaries of the privileges of race and class. At the same time, sick building syndrome expressed the sense that privilege was imperfect, even threatened. Chemical dangers could not be cordoned off to out-of-the-way neighborhoods or distant countries; on the contrary, they lurked nearby in the most unexpected places. The very materials and technologies of postwar comfort and success might themselves be sources of subtle and stealthy chemical exposure. Even the most innocuous products could contribute to the constant background of chemical stimuli.

At mid century, glass-box architecture was accompanied by rhapsodic optimism. Yet during the 1970s, a resurgent feminism and a newly articulated environmentalism spawned an office-workers movement that made occupational health, and particularly chemical exposures, one of its concerns. Office workers gathered complaints about their workplace with simple photocopied questionnaires. Surveys collected the many ways relatively privileged people understood their health as a reaction to possibly hidden chemical dangers in their daily environment. Bodies signaled the possible presence of hazards through common, minor ailments such as headaches and rarer, serious diseases such as cancer. The new physical space of office buildings, combined with anxiety over the buildup of tiny toxic hazards, led to protests that in turn triggered government investigations of office buildings.

Occupational health investigators who traditionally investigated factories or acute chemical spills—engineers, toxicologists, and industrial hygienists—were now called on to inspect nonindustrial, seemingly comfortable office buildings. Once in office buildings, their equipment almost never registered a chemical exposure. No overpopulous molecule, no errant fume, no physical cause could be found. To make matters more complicated, complaining office workers did not even share a common disease, which could then be tracked to an offending germ.

Instead, investigators were confronted with a messy litany of runny noses, scratchy rashes, endless fatigue, burning inhalations, and queasy stomachs. In the early 1980s, these occupational health events acquired the name *sick building syndrome*.

What exactly the name referred to, or if it even referred to anything, was highly contested. In the absence of a definitive cause, some experts claimed that women, who made up the vast majority of office workers, were experiencing "mass hysteria" triggered by stress and facilitated by a feminine coping style or even by menstrual irregularities. Workers' compensation administrators and health insurance companies, in turn, balked at covering a health problem that could not be made to fit traditional explanations. Despite such hesitation, worker protests kept repeating and proliferating during the 1990s, making sick buildings one of the most common types of occupational health investigations in the United States during that decade. A new kind of chemical exposure—indoor pollution—had been identified, not from a discovery in a medical laboratory or clinic but from changes in the ways ordinary people created knowledge about and experienced their everyday environment.[1] Yet not everyone believed that indoor pollution was a real menace. Some scientists, environmentalists, and doctors, bolstered by representatives from chemical manufacturers, held that slight exposures emanating from the commodities of daily life were not a significant worry. In contrast, other scientists, doctors, and activists, joined by experts sponsored by the tobacco industry, held that indoor pollution was in fact a significant worry, perhaps even more so than industrial pollution. They argued that tiny exposures accumulated in otherwise unremarkable interiors and that these exposures, in their sheer multitude, were impossible to untangle from their specific sources. Thus no single product or company could be blamed. Vapors seeped from the abundant and ubiquitous accoutrements of comfortable postwar culture. Was it the new carpet at work? Or the particle board cabinets at home?

As a history of the inside of ordinary office buildings in the twentieth century written at the opening of the twenty-first, this book seeks to capture the ways relatively privileged twentieth-century Americans resided in a world filled with possible chemical exposure. Indoor exposures were possible because the material landscape of privilege had changed in the twentieth century. Yet, unlike the nineteenth century, indoor spaces were no longer filled with smoke and soot from heating, lighting, and cooking flames; they were no longer coated with lead-based paints, no longer lacking in basic plumbing that could flush away organic waste. Of course, even before the twentieth century the objects and materials that formed and populated interiors could emit potentially toxic molecules. In fact, in many ways the indoors had dramatically improved. So why in the late twentieth century did indoor chemical exposures become a serious environmental health concern? Indoor pollution became not just materially present but also a perceptible, definable, knowable object that both experts and laypeople sought to detect and alter.

Historians of medicine have paid important and considerable attention to how microbes have become objects of fear, management, and regulation since the advent of germ theory, shaping the habits of popular culture as well as the practice of medicine for over a century.[2] We understand far less about how chemical exposures similarly came to populate the twentieth-century world as cultural objects of attention and practice. Sick building syndrome exemplifies the ways exposures became part of everyday American life.

The historical scholarship concerning chemical exposures has tended to concentrate on the production of industrial pollution, tracking the uneven distribution of environmental hazards across class and race lines. The history of nonindustrial pollution in comparison, for which there is almost no scholarship, brings into focus how chemical exposures and environmental hazards were also gendered. Office buildings in the twentieth century were deeply gendered spaces: they had become sites for the articulation of a gendered division of labor and a landscape of privilege in which most menial office work was designated a kind of "women's work." Unlike the experts called to investigate their unrest, the bulk of low-status office workers were women with aspirations of benefiting from the privilege and safety of nonindustrial work. Beginning in the 1970s and throughout the 1980s—the decades when sick building syndrome erupted—office workers could draw on resurgent feminisms to challenge this gendered division of labor. Thus, protests over the environmental conditions in nonindustrial workplaces happened contemporaneously with accusations of gender oppression and clashes over women's appropriate place.

In debates between experts over the reality of sick building syndrome, the fact that women made up the majority of complainants opened up the possibility of using the diagnosis of hysteria to explain worker unrest. For complainants themselves, practices of feminist organizing, as well as gendered performances of health care and detailed empathetic attention, could be drawn on to produce counter-narratives that argued for the reality of oppressive and unsafe conditions. Whether in ventilation engineering, office management, or worker activism, gender was a generative ingredient in the physical arrangements of the built environment, in the kinds of authority marshaled in debates, and in the explanations used to argue for the existence or nonexistence of chemical injury. This book highlights the versatile and volatile work of gender in twentieth-century practices of rendering environmental health hazards perceptible and knowable. In the 1980s, gender and chemical exposures both generated controversy and uncertainty.

Sick building syndrome was a postmodern health problem, in form as well as time. Not only did it emerge in the information workplaces of the late twentieth century, its definitions encapsulated a conundrum that was postmodern in form: What are we to make of an object with no essence? As a syndrome, it was recognized only as a constellation of symptoms, not by an underlying mechanism.[3] A typical definition of sick building syndrome depicted it as a *diversity* of ill health effects, mostly minor and associated with a building, for which *no specific cause* was found. Difference expressed itself in workers' health complaints and in each building's complex conditions. Though many investigators and labor activists hoped that a cause would someday be found, sick building syndrome came to be defined formally through its very lack of causal explanation. In fact, once a specific exposure was detected, an episode was no longer diagnosed as a sick building.

Sick building syndrome was thus a doubly troublesome phenomenon to affirm: it was found in spaces expected to be safe, even comfortable, and it was nonspecific and multiple both in its cause and expression. The words "sick building" signaled a confusion of boundaries between buildings and the bodies in them—how can a building be sick?—and an attempt to make sense of complexity by making buildings the unit of analysis. It was the mantra "in the building . . . in the building," repeated in cities across the country, that lent sick building syndrome its coherence.

Most discussions in the late twentieth century of sick buildings, and transient or low-level exposures more generally, were caught in a debate about the very existence of these events: Were they real or not? Did a toxic exposure occur or not? The controversies around the "reality" of sick buildings provided me, as a historian, with an opportunity to study how laypeople and experts have struggled to prove or disprove an environmental health problem. In this book, I do not employ history to judge in favor of one side or the other. Nor do I set out to explain sick building syndrome as the history of an idea. Such analyses can too easily be interpreted as arguing that indoor chemical exposures were and are not "real." They can be too easily used against current claims of chemical injury, too easily plugged into antilabor arguments that assert sick building syndrome was simply a phantasm of illness, that it was only the medicalization of labor problems by disgruntled and hysterical women. Writing about the historicity of chemical exposures in the recent past is treacherous when one's arguments are always in danger of being reframed as affirming the unreality of exposures.

In this book, then, I take a step back from this controversy by using sick building syndrome as an entry point into historicizing the practices by which chemical exposures were granted or not granted existence. That is, I am concerned with how exposures were *materialized*.[4] Though an empirical study of the past, this is not a straightforward chronological account of the rise of sick building syndrome; instead it is a juxtaposition of histories, each delineating how an expert or lay tradition made chemical exposures perceptible or imperceptible, existent or nonexistent. Instead of resolving the factualness or fallacy of any given case of exposure, I am concerned with historicizing the techniques through which "exposure," as an effect between buildings and bodies, became a phenomenon people could say, feel, and do something about. Moreover, I want to understand the history of how chemical exposures were not only materialized but materialized as *uncertain* events. How were exposures imbued with uncertainty? This book treats these as historical questions that necessitate thinking about the historical ontology of exposures.

Historical ontology is a term developed by historians and philosophers of science to describe historical accounts of how objects, such as germs, immune systems, subatomic particles, diseases, and so on, came into being as recognizable objects via historically specific circumstances.[5] Studies of historical ontology typically hold that what counts as truth is the result of historically specific practices of truth-telling—laboratory techniques, instruments, methods of observing, modes of calculating, regimes of classification, and so on—and, importantly, that the objects that are apprehended through that truth-telling are also historical.[6]

Examining the history of how objects came into being does not imply a claim that the world only affects us in ways that humans can perceive. Chemical exposures do *not* only happen when we know about them. Instead, attention to historical ontology underlines that it was only in the eighteenth century, when humans found ways to detect and manipulate entities called molecules, that we could assert that molecules had always existed even before we knew about them. Now that we have molecules we need them and do things with them; they are things we cannot live without. Molecules now have atoms, bonds, polymers, and other properties that we study, manipulate, and even manufacture. At the same time, attending to historical ontology allows the possibility that in the future other objects and properties that do not exist for us now may come into being for us, and in doing so perhaps even make the object "molecule" a less useful description for truth-telling. Thus, attending to the historical quality of existence is a way to hold onto the concreteness of things in the world in a given moment, while at the same time allowing for the possibility that other, yet undeveloped, ways of registering, slicing up, and bringing into being the complexity of the world are, were, and will be made possible by new instruments, techniques, social movements, and so on.

This book makes two main arguments about the historical ontology of chemical exposures. First, I argue that exposures were brought into existence in multiple, often conflicting circumstances—the result of not just specific environments but also new arrangements of technologies and practices through which laypeople, scientists, and corporate experts apprehended the health effects of buildings on bodies.[7] Second, I argue that any given way of materializing chemical exposures as perceptible and real also sets the terms of what was imperceptible and unreal. Indoor chemical exposures, I argue, came into being through multiple histories that did not all agree on the terms by which an exposure could be shown to have happened or not.[8]

Invisible to our eyes, chemicals wafting from carpet, ink, and adhesive are starring protagonists in the story of sick building syndrome. Environmental historians and historians of science have often debated how best to include nonhuman actors—such as buildings or molecules—in

historical accounts.[9] Environmental historians have included mos-
quitoes, prairie grass, weather, geological processes, and microbes as
actors that have had important, often deadly, consequences for human
history. To grant such actors specific agency in their narratives, environmental historians have tended to turn to contemporary scientific findings in order to characterize their actors' qualities, habits, and consequences. When it comes to chemical exposures, however, contemporary
scientific findings, often originating in corporate laboratories, are contested by other communities of experts or by laypeople claiming to suffer chemical injury. The science on chemical exposures is simply unreli-
able by our contemporary standards of scientific truth. Moreover, no
scientific studies exist for a vast number of chemicals used in industry.
Thus there is a dual uncertainty when it comes to chemical exposures:
first, any incidence of chemical exposure is difficult to pinpoint, even
with scientific best efforts, because of the complexity of the phenomenon itself; second, contemporary experts disagree about the import and
even the existence of widespread, low-level exposures. This dual uncertainty is thus an important problematic for environmental historians,
prompting increased attention to questions of how "unknowing," ignorance, and imperception were not just accidentally but purposefully
generated in the history of knowledge practices.[10]

Perceptibility and imperceptibility are this book's central concerns.
Not only was the ability to register chemical exposures as existent the
result of specific historical practices and technologies, but so too was the
inability to register them. The history of how objects were rendered
perceptible was in the same gesture intrinsically linked to a delineation
of what was imperceptible.[11] The history of how things come to exist is
intrinsically linked to the history of how things come not to exist, or
come to exist only with uncertainty or partially. In other words, seeing
necessitates the designation of the unseeable, knowing the unknowable,
and so on. *Domains of imperceptibility* were the inevitable results of the
tangible ways scientists and laypeople came to render chemical exposures measurable, quantifiable, assessable, and knowable in some ways
and not others.[12]

Domains of imperceptibility were produced by limits in the capacities
of knowledge practices, limits that were inevitable—every discipline of
knowledge studies some things and not others; every scientific instrument can detect some things and not others; every experiment includes

some variables and not others. These material limits in knowledge production were and still are at stake in debates over the existence of chemical exposures. By juxtaposing different, sometimes conflicting traditions of knowledge production—toxicology with popular epidemiology, for example—one can throw limits into relief. I have layered and contrasted a select, and by no means exhaustive, set of histories in which scientific disciplines and lay communities rendered chemical exposures as events that one could or could not do something about. I will call the way a discipline or epistemological tradition perceives and does not perceive the world its *regime of perceptibility*.[13]

Chemical exposures are contentious events. They involve litigation, blame, neglect, and suffering. Chemical corporations, tobacco companies, manufacturers, and employers, as well as government administrations with antiregulation ideologies, have been deeply invested in producing science that minimizes or denies exposures. Such actors have developed techniques that maintain chemical exposure and their health effects as uncertain, that is, as events that one cannot do something about. Over the course of the twentieth century imperceptibility itself became a quality that could be produced through the design of experiments or monitoring equipment in order to render claims of chemical exposures uncertain. Other groups of laypeople and experts have nonetheless developed their own practices and technologies to produce evidence for the reality of harmful chemical exposures. Through their efforts domains of imperceptibility have become populated with all sorts of qualities, such as multiplicity, nonspecificity, complexity, and so on.

It is possible to track the production of imperceptibility because what was generated as imperceptible in one place could be generated as perceptible elsewhere. It is precisely by tracing the confluence of different histories for apprehending office buildings that I have tried to throw domains of imperceptibility into relief. I show that imperceptibility was not only accidentally and inevitably produced, it was also at times purposefully generated and maintained, particularly, but not exclusively, by industry-sponsored science. In either case, this book suggests regimes of perceptibility actively participated in making chemical exposures the phenomena they are today. In order to throw imperceptibility into relief through juxtaposition, this book makes a second argument about the historical ontology of exposures: objects are many things at once.

Multiplicities and Assemblages

A useful way to begin thinking about the historicity of chemical exposures in ordinary buildings, like the one you may be sitting in right
now, is to see them as one of the ways buildings are physically connected
to bodies. We can then ask about the buildings themselves. What is an
office building? It is a real estate venture, built to maximize the developer's profit. And at the same time, a building has a mechanical
physicality; it is a structure of steel and concrete, walls and ventilation
ducts that mechanically delivers an indoor atmosphere. It is a structure
for efficiently organizing the work of late capitalism, giving material
form to economy, and dividing people into function and rank. Its potted
plants, logos, and design are symbols of a company's prestige. Office
buildings are repetitious, using the same mass-produced elements over
and over, so that one becomes disoriented in a built space that seems to
be the same no matter what the particularities of its location. Once an
office building is launched into the world, it becomes its own unique
hive of activity, bringing people together, spawning meetings, hierarchies, friendships, and sexual encounters both wanted and unwanted,
worn out in one area and neglected in another. There is this office
building I work in, and the one I used to work in, and the one next door,
and . . . and. . . . In short, office buildings, like all objects, are multiplicities composed of many histories, of "ands," that link in ways intended and unintended, drawing out some attributes and not others,
thereby setting the conditions of possibility for buildings.[14]

  The multiplicitous building connects with the bodies inside in myriad
ways: guiding movement through space, indicating appropriate behaviors, demarcating privilege, segregating by race and gender. The first
refinement of my question, then, is how did buildings, in all their concrete multiplicity, affect the health of bodies? Not just any bodies, but the
bodies of women office workers in the late twentieth century, who numerically predominated in the grunt labor of American information
work. Which is not to say that they were only laboring bodies; they were
also gendered and raced bodies dressed in middle-class clothes, dif-
ferentiating themselves from factory workers. Which is not to say bodies
were only social; they were also organic, composed of flesh and bone,
organ systems, biochemical cycles, and immunological reactions, an
organic body deciphered and anatomized by the practice of biomedicine,

that in turn drew on instruments, laboratories, and clinical practices to apprehend and monitor sickness and health. All of this is to say that bodies, like buildings, can concretely be many things at once—they are also multiplicities. Instead of a simple *is*, they are made possible by *and*s: woman and worker and flesh and . . . and . . . and. . . . Put simply, objects are constituted through their manifold material relationships, and these relationships have different histories.[15] This is not to say that a sum total of *and*s can add up to a full understanding of a building. Multiplicities are not like the interlocking pieces of a jigsaw puzzle, which fit together to reveal a single picture. Histories may overlap and contradict each other, have varying intensities, durations, and stabilities. Instead of asking, What *is* a building? I will be asking, What are its *and*s? What did its historical relations make possible?

Buildings and bodies were often connected. A building was built with bodies in mind; it became a prosthesis of the body, extending its functions. The body, in turn, became a mobile part of the building; it was vulnerable without the shelter of the building, which supplied the milieu that organized its movements. Buildings and bodies were caught up in one another, sharing themselves in each other's conditions of possibilities, tracing each other's contours.[16] They were in a relationship of mutual presupposition, a mutual capture in which they altered one another. Each was an integral element in the chains of "ands" that made up the other. A building is derelict without bodies inhabiting it. It is very difficult to be a body without the shelter of a building.

I use the term *assemblage* to describe the historically specific patterns through which buildings and bodies were connected, or assembled, to each other and to the objects and practices around them.[17] I define "assemblage" as an arrangement of discourses, objects, practices, and subject positions that work together within a particular discipline or knowledge tradition. It is not the list of elements that make an assemblage consequential, it is what they made possible by the ways they articulated each other.[18] In describing the assemblages within different traditions of knowledge production, I have tried to attend to how arrangements of words, things, practices and people drew out and made perceptible specific qualities, capacities, and possibilities for buildings and bodies. In other words, how an assemblage created a regime of perceptibility.

To get at a given assemblage, I have "cracked open" the archive of technical guides, minutes of meetings, questionnaires, instruments, and body parts that made up a scientific discipline or lay epistemological tradition. By cracking open, I am looking for an abstract regularity to the way objects, subjects, practices, and words articulated each other. What I am trying to describe by writing about assemblages are historical *regularities*.[19] Regularities are not simply a set of objects or phrases that appear often in the historical record. What I am calling regularities are not hidden, though historical actors may not necessarily recognize them. Regularities are the pattern of arrangement that is repeated, congealed, and constitutive of a scientific discipline or epistemological tradition. I use the abstraction of the assemblage as a means to investigate these congealed conditions of possibility for an archive, what was and was not sayable, perceivable, doable, natural, possible, and so on about buildings and chemical exposures in a particular historical circumstance. To get at these regularities, I examined archives belonging to ventilation engineering, feminist labor activism, and toxicology (to name a few examples) and sought to describe the assemblage of practices, technologies, and words that governed what was historically possible.

I find the idea of the assemblage a very useful concept to talk about the historically specific ways chemical exposures were apprehended, that is, became events that one could or could not say something and do something about. When I used the concept of assemblage, it became clearer to me that objects existed by virtue of their historically specific and yet very tangible and material circumstances. Assemblages are formed of organic and inorganic objects, technologies, bodies, and architecture, and not just of words. In this way, I wish to convey that chemical exposures in the twentieth century were materialized as events with particular kinds of qualities—and not others—by virtue of concrete technical and social arrangements. I therefore use the concept of the assemblage to describe the material and yet relational way things came to matter. An assemblage materializes an object by placing it in a specific social and technical constellation, making it perceptible, outlining form, drawing out possibilities and investing meanings by virtue of its linkages, effects, and relationships. Or conversely, by ordering an object in an assemblage, that object could be disinvested of qualities, capacities, and possibilities, thereby becoming dematerialized, even deemed nonexistent.

Buildings and bodies were called into being in as many ways as there were assemblages that seized them. A building could be part of both an assemblage of ventilation systems, engineers, and standardization, *and* an assemblage of office work, workers, and occupational health problems. A body could be part of both an assemblage of doctors, insurance companies, and diseases, *and* an assemblage of feminism, consciousness-raising, and personal experience. This is what makes them multiplicities. When I traced any given assemblage by following its history and asking how it works, I found out that each element itself already had many other histories running through it. Our interior landscapes are embedded in a multitude of histories that do not necessarily sit well with each other. Objects or qualities vital in one assemblage may not be relevant in another. One assemblage may bring into being what another disavows or simply does not register. It is precisely by understanding sick buildings as materialized in the encounter of disciplinarily specific assemblages (from engineering, management, toxicology, feminism, popular epidemiology, cybernetics, etc.) that I hope to better understand not only how chemical exposures became part of everyday privileged American culture, but also how chemical exposures became quintessentially uncertain events.

Office workers, thus, did not magically make sick building syndrome out of thin air—poof, now there is an object where before there was nothing.[20] It is not so easy to materialize a new object. First, despite what we might wish, the world is not passive and cannot be made to work in whatever way we might hope. Objects were successfully materialized when they captured some of the potentialities and possibilities in our world. Moreover, once materialized, objects were not neutral. They resisted in the manner with which they had already become present. Thus, materializations are always *rematerializations*.[21] Such rematerialization can sometimes be a form of resistance, not in the sense of liberation but in the sense of maintaining or producing possibilities counter to or cutting across dominant ways of apprehending reality.[22] Or an encounter can result in a dematerialization, in which what is done in one assemblage is actively undone in another.

This book tries to show in empirical detail how sick buildings were formed by different, often conflicting, histories that remade and sometimes undid the "reality" of chemical exposures. Sick buildings existed in between office worker protests, feminism, ventilation engineering, toxicology, popular epidemiology, corporate science, and ecology. Many different ways of connecting buildings and bodies seized on seemingly safe workplaces, and no two seized it in quite the same way. It was at this intersection of making and unmaking that indoor chemical exposures became events about which little could be asserted with certainty. At stake in writing a history of the contested reality of chemical exposures is the historicity of what counts as real, of what did and did not matter. To do this, I have conveyed matter, not in terms of a prior thingness but rather in terms of the processes of history, concrete social and technical arrangements and the effects of power—hence my use of the verb *materialize*. At the same time, and like most historians of science, I insist on the importance of environmental chambers, building materials, molecules, questionnaires, immune systems, and other tangible agents as physical actors in this process.

Sick building syndrome as a topic necessitated thinking about the relationship between history, materiality, and uncertainty. There is a materiality about sickness that is very difficult, and indeed dangerous, to deny. In debates about sick building syndrome in the recent past, medical and environmental experts were the ones most often claiming that sick building syndrome was not real, while workers were more likely to say it was. In order to understand the coming into being of indoor chemical exposures, then, I had to examine lay knowledge practices along with scientific ones. Chemical exposures, moreover, remain notoriously difficult events to prove. The subject itself both provoked questions of materiality and imperceptibility and made them unavoidable.

The chapters that make up this book are about historical regularities, not explanations of specific events. My narratives are abstractions of the regularities I encountered in my empirical research. Yet there is a contradiction buried deep in my methods: I was trying to explain a tangle clearly. In trying to be clear, I fear my narratives are too rigid and simple, leaving out much of the messiness. In trying to diagram the overwhelming histories about buildings and chemical exposures, I have stressed the structure over the confusion. Despite this limitation, I hope that the reader will be able imagine how these other words, objects, and subjects could also be exploded into multiplicities and how they, too, are contentiously rematerialized.

The book nonetheless remains an empirical investigation into the past of an important subject—chemical exposures. I have only gone to such lengths to think about materiality and history because I have taken very seriously the problem of writing a history of the twentieth century's polluted backdrop and its largely unregistered health effects.[23] It is in this spirit that I have used the terms *assemblages, materialization,* and *regimes of perceptibility,* not just as colorful speech but as means of interrogating a problem. I have used the terms as my toolbox, and I try to make them do useful intellectual work. I have no illusion that my methodological toolbox forms an architecture of propositions that finally solves the problem of the relationship between history and materiality or the uncertainty of chemical exposures. A book is also an assemblage, of words, paper, and reader, and I invite you to make use of it as you will.

Map

Though they can be read separately, together the chapters in this book operate as a single argument about the historicity, multiplicity, and imperceptibility of chemical exposures. Each chapter cracks open the practices through which a discipline or epistemological tradition connected buildings and bodies. Most chapters emphasize a disciplinary assemblage of objects, practices, and discourses and the way that assemblage materialized bodies and building and thus rendered chemical exposures perceptible and imperceptible. Some technologies and practices, such as environmental chambers and surveys, reappear in different chapters, so that in reading the book as a whole one might see how these technologies performed differently in various historical circumstances.

Chapter 1 cracks open ventilation engineering and the experiments that set the criteria for the construction of mid-century buildings as machines that provided indoor weather. By examining the assemblage by which ventilation standards were established in the interwar years, I argue that building-machines generated a standardized "comfort" that required a standardized body, while at the same time leaving chemical attributes of the indoor atmosphere as outside of mechanical control, irrelevant to comfort, and imperceptible. How work was organized in office buildings, from Taylorism to cybernetics, is the subject of chapter 2, which examines how distributions of desks, pathways of paper, and the exertion of equipment formed tightly knit material and social assemblages for choreographing the labor of office workers. This chapter outlines the history of the material organization of office work and the ways the exercise of power depended on not only gendered and classed subjects but also machined subjects. By this I mean the way bodies were materialized as parts within a larger corporate apparatus. I argue that by the 1970s the material organization of office work encompassed a growing tension between its comfortable and middle-class milieu and the actual status of most office workers. Chapter 3 traces the history of the women's office worker movement in the 1970s and 1980s, examining how it rematerialized the comfortable office as a site of gender oppression, and then toxic exposure, that was dispersed in the minutiae of office work. This chapter argues that the office worker movement used surveys to gather "experience" that in turn materialized office buildings as dangerous locations, setting the stage for the sick building episodes. Moreover, the way the movement rematerialized toxicity rendered specific causal narratives untenable.

In chapter 4, the book turns to the practices through which sick buildings themselves were investigated. The methods of industrial hygienists and toxicologists, which had developed for the study of acute industrial exposures in the first half of the century, are contrasted with the methods of the social survey movement and later popular epidemiological practices of toxic waste activists. This chapter situates sick building syndrome in the clash between two different domains of imperceptibility produced by toxicology and popular epidemiology.

The racialization of privilege and imperceptibility is the subject of chapter 5, which takes as its case study activism by EPA scientists in the 1980s and their efforts to define the EPA headquarters as a sick building. This chapter links the invisibility of racialized distributions of environmental privilege to its benefactors with ways of explaining the presence of chemical exposures in buildings. Chapter 6 turns our attention to the emergence of privately contracted building investigators in the 1990s and the practice of building ecology. It argues that system ecology's emphasis on management, relationships, and multiplicities facilitated taking a managerial approach to indoor chemical exposures as well as assisting the antiregulatory politics of the tobacco industry. By looking at how multiplicity was made a crucial quality of ecologies and at the same time used to shore up imperceptibility and unaccountability to the chemically injured, this chapter seeks to problematize any uncritical celebration of multiplicity.

The book's seventh and final chapter looks at the history of multiple chemical sensitivity (MCS), a controversial illness associated with indoor pollution in the late twentieth century. This chapter examines the coping strategies of people whose bodies reacted to the indoor environment in ways unacceptable to dominant medicine. It argues that domains of imperceptibility, unintelligibility, and impossibility can nonetheless be densely populated. I trace how chemically injured people practiced experimental divestments and reinvestments in order to bring intelligibility to their bodies and create safe spaces in which to live. I argue that this experimentation was necessary to materialize MCS from below and at the same time dangerous in its reification of unintelligibility to others.

This book sets out to show that sick building syndrome and chemical exposures cannot be adequately understood by answering the question, "Is it real or not?" The chapters' narratives accumulate to argue that the very terms of this question can be understood as an effect of historical processes. Exposures are made to matter.

Man in a Box
Building-Machines and the Science of Comfort

[1] **Crack open an office building** constructed from the late twentieth century and you will find a machine. Behind glass and concrete, behind suspended ceilings and drywall were the building's guts: aluminum ducts worming through dense pink insulation, crisscrossed wires delivering electrical signals, boilers burbling in basements, droning fans caged by grates. Office buildings in the late twentieth century were machines engineered to control the *indoor climate*. They were machines designed to encourage the buzz of "information" work inside and to produce a clean, orderly corporate world sealed off from both the polluted outdoors and the dangerous factory floor.

Office buildings were not just luxurious spaces for the American managerial class; they were also constructed to promote the efficient labor of the droves of mostly women in the office's lower ranks. Perceptions about the physiological needs of these laborers were built into the very pipes and ducts of office buildings. Not simply a pleasant and passive backdrop, the office building's cool, comfortable air was the material manifestation of a historically specific, gendered, and raced way of apprehending the relationship between office workers' bodies and the spaces that ordered their labor. More specifically, inscribed into the humidifiers and thermostats was a mechanistic and "modernist" way of assembling bodies and buildings together, a formula set in the interwar years. It was a relatively simple assemblage, shaped by the reductionism of that era, and thus the building-as-machine is a useful history to crack open first. While at initial glance an arcane topic, the history of ventilation engineering is installed in virtually every building constructed in the late-twentieth-century United States.[1] Sitting in your office, the university library, or even your home, you feel this history every day.

Man in a Box

Imagine a ventilation engineering laboratory in the years between the world wars, when standardization signaled the height of scientism. The focal point of the lab was the "psychrometric room," a small square side room separated off from the rest of the lab to form an environmental chamber.[2] The chamber was sealed airtight. It was an empty box (see the "air conditioning room" in Fig. 1).

Inside the box, young white men, mostly engineering students, sometimes stripped to underwear, repetitively lifted light weights. Outside the chamber, the researchers, sleeves rolled, used sensitive instruments such as the hot-wire anemometer and the whirled psychrometer to monitor the interior atmosphere.[3] They used anal thermometers and odor scales to probe their subjects' physiological responses to mechanically generated climates. These older white men, university professors or presidents of lucrative air-conditioning businesses (such as the Carrier Air Conditioning Corporation), were members of the American Society for Heating and Ventilation Engineers (ASHVE). One of the ASHVE's most exalted projects was undertaken by the Research Technical Advisory Committee on Physiological Reactions, which experimentally studied how to mechanically fabricate an indoor climate for human comfort.[4] In the 1920s, their research into human comfort and artificial environments commanded lab space at Harvard and Yale, gained government support at the U.S. Bureau of Mines, and attracted distinguished researchers, such as Wallis Carrier, the "father of air conditioning," C.-E. A. Winslow, the respected editor of the *American Journal of Public Health*, and Constantine Yaglou and Philip Drinker, professors in Harvard's Department of Industrial Hygiene.[5] Studying men in boxes (and boxers) was their means of scientifically articulating an "optimum" indoor climate for nonindustrial buildings of all sorts, but especially office buildings, whose owners were among their biggest customers. They were searching for a *universal* indoor climatic standard that could be manufactured within any building, anywhere—what the architect Le Corbusier called "respiration exact," but what ASHVE engineers more prosaically termed "the comfort zone."

What qualities made up "comfort" in the great indoors of the interwar years? What qualities were inserted into the empty box? ASHVE researchers concentrated on just three: temperature, humidity, and air-

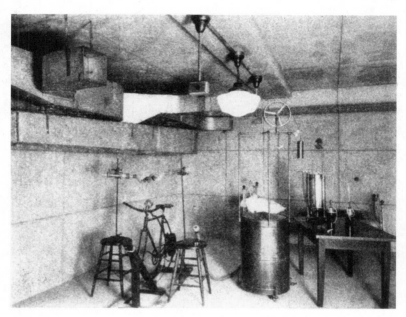

Figure 1. The "air conditioning room" of the Laboratory of Ventilation and Illumination at the Harvard School of Public Health in 1924. In this sealed cement room, insulated with two inches of cork, temperature, humidity, and airflow were mechanically controlled. Next door in the "temperature control room," the scientists calibrated and controlled the climate conditions and communicated to subjects with wires, bell, and a telephone. The physiological reactions of test subjects were recorded at various levels of exertion, such as riding a stationary bicycle or lifting weights, to simulate labor. From Drinker, "Laboratories of Ventilation."

flow.[6] In a self-referential circle, these researchers sought to measure comfort only in terms of those attributes of air altered by the ventilation technologies their companies already manufactured. Temperature had long been alterable upward with steam radiators or heated forced air; airflow with fans and ducts. The ability to mechanically alter humidity, called "air conditioning," was relatively new in the early twentieth century, having first been developed for industrial processes and only in this period extended to "comfort cooling."[7] Other qualities, such as the molecular composition of air or the microbes that floated within it, remained undetected by ASHVE's experimental setup. What was uncontrolled and undetected in the box remained irrelevant to their project of comfort and in practice resided in the realm of imperceptibility. Only temperature, humidity, and airflow, and not other attributes, were materialized by modern ventilation engineering.

Yet in the recent past, before engineers-turned-merchants hawked air conditioners, other qualities had populated indoor air. Ventilation engineers had previously promoted the mechanical supply of "fresh air" in the name of healthfulness, not comfort. The fight against foul air, excess carbon dioxide, and miasma (disease-causing air emanating from organic matter, such as filthy rivers, waste piles, and human bodies) had allied ventilation engineers with public health reformers, called sanitarians, who sought to improve the living conditions of the worthy laboring poor by constructing sewers, treating drinking water, and legislating standards for fresh air in tenements, schools, and factories.[8] "Ventilation comes next to godliness," preached one such reform-minded engineer.[9] But foul air also plagued the middle classes, who commonly observed that stale air, while not deadly as in tenements, lowered the body's vigor, causing "dullness, headache, sleepiness, fainting, nausea, and the like."[10] Both miasma and excess carbon dioxide were exuded from people's bodies. The engineering solution to these worrisome exhalations was dilution of "stale air" with "fresh air" from the outside. For the urban middle class, concern over stale air was shaped by a class anxiety over the close proximity of the "great unwashed" in tight urban spaces.[11] By the mid-twentieth century, it would be this white middle class whose built environment benefited most from sanitarian services.[12]

At its most economical and widely practiced in the nineteenth and early twentieth centuries, ventilation was simply opening windows. In contrast to this commonsense provision of fresh air, the emerging professional field of ventilation engineering solicited its business by arguing that only machines could reliably and precisely deliver fresh air in the volume and quality necessary to guarantee healthfulness. Yet, just as ventilation engineers were making their pitch, the theories that validated the need for fresh air fell out of favor. Quickly in the twentieth century, miasma was made an outdated concept by germ theory, just as the carbon dioxide theory of stale air was also experimentally overturned.[13] By 1923, the influential New York City Commission on Ventilation vehemently called into question the previous century's fervor—and expenditure—for "fresh air."[14] There was simply little scientific or public consensus about what made air healthful, or even whether mechanical air supplies were superior to natural ones.

In the interwar years, moreover, the indoor environment in which the professional middle class dwelt and labored had materially changed from the conditions that had inspired public health reformer's zeal for fresh air. Office buildings were heated with steam radiators, not coal, and were supplied with electricity that powered lighting and fans, thereby clearing the indoor air of its former smoke and soot.[15] In the skyscrapers that now spiked downtowns, mechanical services of pipes, elevators, and wiring were modern engineering feats in themselves. Outside, downtown streets were crowded and polluted—there was less "fresh air" for ventilation to bring in.

Office buildings with mechanical ventilation now could become havens from the people and pollution out on the sidewalk. "Man-made weather," so ventilation engineers began to argue, could shelter the privileged from the stenches and unsavory minglings of urban civilization and the corporeal discomforts of fickle natural weather. In the 1920s, with declining support for the old ideology of fresh air, ASHVE engineers began searching for new means to secure their livelihood and articulate their work. Through their efforts the indoor environment was imbued with the virtue of "comfort" (not health), an attribute they sought to experimentally qualify and mechanically generate. "Comfort" as an attribute invested with scientism also had the asset of being a luxury of wealth. By providing comfort, ventilation engineering set out to construct a new environmental norm for privileged citizens. Once a norm of privilege, the mere provision of widespread mechanical ventilation could signal an escape into privilege for the masses—the escapist spaces of movie theaters were the mass public's first exposure to the ephemeral effects of cool. Selling comfort through science became the interwar ventilation engineer's trade.

Beginning in 1919, the central technical problem of the ASHVE research program was to specify a point of universal comfort by calibrating the triumvirate of temperature, humidity, and airflow within environmental chambers. Crack open this experimental setup and one can find an assemblage within the discipline of ventilation engineering that gave indoor comfort its distinctive form.

I use the term *assemblage* to describe the technical and social constellation of words, things, practices, and people that governed what was possible in a given discipline. Interwar ventilation developed at its heart a configuration of subject positions, objects, practices, and discourses that articulated one another and that, by working together, drew out specific capacities and qualities for buildings, their inhabitants, and the researchers studying them. Such knowledge-producing assemblages allowed the apprehension of some stimuli and not others. Any method of perception was materially constrained, such as by employing only part of the spectrum of light waves (human eyes are different from bee eyes) or by only focusing on objects of a certain size (microscopes vs. telescopes) or by only registering phenomena occurring at certain speeds and not others (such as the slowness of geological time). Perception always involves disengaging from a broader field of possibilities for the sake of focusing on, isolating, and rendering intelligible a more narrowly delineated set of qualities.[16] I call the regular and sedimented contours of perception and imperception produced within a disciplinary or epistemological tradition its "regimes of perceptibility."

Regimes of perceptibility are about more than just what we can see. As regimes, they were often understood by the historical actors employing them as natural or inevitable outcomes of social and technical arrangements. Produced by assemblages that are anchored in material culture, regimes of perceptibility establish what phenomena become perceptible, and thus what phenomena come into being for us, giving objects boundaries and imbuing them with qualities. Regimes of perceptibility populate our world with some objects and not others, and they allow certain actions to be performed on those objects. The experimental setup in ASHVE's environmental chamber relied on an assemblage that produced just such a regime of perceptibility for the apprehension of the effects of buildings on bodies in terms of "comfort."

The assemblage of interwar ventilation engineering began with an empty box. It was a tabula rasa into which measurable variables could be inserted under controlled circumstances and their effects untangled and extracted from the messy politics and confounding influences of actual workplaces. While the environmental chamber stood in for the building, the experimental subjects within—usually young, white, male engineering students—stood in for office workers. Their mild physical activities, such as methodically pedaling a stationary bike, were held as abstract equivalents to the labor expended working on light office machinery: labor in a box. The human body itself, moreover, was to be regarded as a machine. As one ventilation engineer explained, bodies could be "regarded as a combination of radiator, thermostat and humidifier."[17] Like other interwar researchers calibrating the efficiency of the laboring body, engineers studied the skin-sealed human motor as they did other machines, by measuring inputs and outputs.[18] The artificial climate made within the environmental chamber was the input. The output was comfortable and productive labor as indicated by such physiological measurements as those of pulse, weight loss, "metabolism" (exhaled breath), and body temperature. Distanced from medical concerns, the body that ventilation engineers investigated was one of skin effects, sweat, and other sensations associated with comfort. "Comfort" was materialized as a neutral atmosphere that least exerted itself on bodies in business dress.

The environment-chamber experiments were a mechanistic microcosm of how building-machines ideally connected to bodies. Buildings could be calibrated to provide inputs that encouraged desirable human outputs. The building-machine presupposed a body-machine, which, like itself, had an optimal level of function. In this way, a machined apprehension of the human body was constructed into buildings. All bodies, no matter how different, strove toward the same ideal of efficiency. Comfort could be universalized. This shared possibility of fleshly comfort, moreover, could be located as a quantifiable combination of just three qualities: temperature, humidity, and airflow. The assemblage of a comfortable human-machine in a box-machine generated combinations of temperature, humidity, and airflow that were then distilled into a statistical representational form, the "comfort zone chart" that could then be built everywhere for everybody. In short, bodies governed by nature's norms could be translated into a universalizable environment.[19]

In practice, the golden point on the graph that identified the optimum climate was charted through measurements largely taken from the bodies of the young, white college men in boxer shorts who acted as the research subjects in their studies, turning a human particular into a universal. In the masculine, homosocial culture of engineering, these were not just any human bodies but the bodies of trustworthy engineers trained in rationality. Measurements were coming from human-motors whose senses were deemed reliable because they were invested with rationality and had bodies that could be coded as "ordinary." In the context of white male privilege in engineering, they were bodies that could be marked as unmarked, as "ordinary," cultureless, raceless, genderless witnesses appropriate to the calculation of an "average" human body—"Man" with a capital M. In full circle, a standardizable environment interpolated a standardizable human. Man in a box translated into a universalized man-made weather precisely because the experiments presupposed a certain kind of humanity. Particular bodies elevated to universals and the mechanically built environment articulated each other, called each other into a particular form. They replicated in a distinctly modernist and straightforward assemblage, one which could generate an interior of universalized "comfort" that optimally would be unnoticeable to its inhabitants, and which in turn was expressed as a standard of privilege.

Though ASHVE engineers held dear their ability to rationally study comfort, the complexity of corporeality resisted being laid bare by instruments alone. By the 1930s, demands in the market turned ASHVE research toward the removal of odor, mostly of the human variety.[20] In places like offices, which were designed to provide a distinguishable middle-class atmosphere and yet allowed men and women clerks to work elbow to elbow, places where secretaries sat within earshot of executives, where janitors swept by managers, where workers of different classes, genders, and sometimes even races increasingly mixed, maintaining an odor-free atmosphere showed that an office building itself could transcend the varieties of its inhabitants and artificially sustain a coding of privilege in its very air. Odorlessness became an essential aspect of unmarkedness, the quintessential attribute of privilege in twentieth-century America.

In their research into odorlessness, ASHVE engineers explicitly placed the human senses in their toolbox among their gauges and psychrometers. The *trained* human nose was praised as the most sensitive of all instruments. The Harvard professor Constantine Yaglou, a leading man behind the comfort zone chart, wrote that "the human nose when properly utilized affords a better criterion of the quality of air in occupied rooms than any of the known physical or chemical tests."[21] Yaglou and his colleagues used men, women, and children from upper and lower classes in these experiments. A variety of kinds of people were needed, not because they had different notions of comfort or sensitivities to smell, but because their bodies produced odors in differing degrees. The turn to subjective sensory assessment exposed the lapses inherent in reducing

the evidence of comfort to instrument gauges. Whether by anal ther-
mometer or sniffing nose, assessments of comfort had to pass through
irrepressible human sensibility. Yet, by emphasizing the trained nose
and numerical odor scales, these engineers tenaciously clung to their
notions of objectivity.

Crack open the building-machine of ventilation engineering. Bodies
were standardizable entities—norms—requiring comfort. Buildings
were boxes into which controllable comfort could be mechanically inserted. What then did ASHVE engineers materialize as they whirled their
psychrometers, sniffed the air, and graphed the results? They were in
search of an enforceable *standard* of comfort. A standard crystallized the
abstract assemblage of Man in a box down to one line of discursive code:
ASHRAE Standard 62 (1938), minimum ventilation of 15 cfm (cubic feet
per minute).[22] Since 1925, the "comfort zone" has been an indoor standard inscribed in the design of mechanical appliances, disseminated in
professional codes and handbooks, guiding the construction of all office
buildings in the United States. A well-constructed building from the interwar years on delivered to its inhabitants a standardized, homogenous,
and unnoticeable environment of temperature, humidity, and airflow.

Corporate Utopias and Total Control

Imagine a corporate headquarters sprawled amid the manicured lawns
of suburban Connecticut in 1958. Each weekday workers pull their aero-
dynamic Chevrolet Impalas and opulent Chrysler Imperials into the
parking lot of the corporate headquarters. As they step out of their cars
and join the flow of people hurrying toward the lobby entrance, they
might wipe sweat from their brows or shiver as they pull their coats
tighter around them, but once they push through the glass revolving
doors their bodies are instantly struck with comfortable, conditioned air.
The building was now a box-machine that could reliably produce an
indoor climate. In the basement catacombs of a mid-century-built corporation sat the heart, or better yet the brain, of the building-machine: the
central control console of the HVAC, the automatic heating, ventilating,
and air conditioning (see Fig. 2). From the lobby to the shoeshine stand
to the typewriter pool, the ducts and fans of the central control console
delivered their standardized environment. In the postwar years the cli-

mate of the ASHVE engineers' experimental chambers became that of large, modernist office buildings. The assemblage had moved from the lab into architecture.

A central control console was a room-sized apparatus covered with flashing lights, large dials, and colored switches; it resembled the design futurism of space vehicles as seen on 1950s television. Such consoles monitored and automated all the fans, circuits, pumps, exhausts, compressors, and air cleaners that architects now incorporated into the physical concrete and steel of buildings. Manned by a single technician, a central control console only required one trained person to monitor dials and push buttons, embodying a fervent mid-century engineering ideology of centralized control, automation, and technocratic utopianism. "Progress in mastering climate and temperature must start with precision control" declares an advertisement in ASHVE's professional journal, as a handsome white engineer in a sleek tailored suit looks off into a futuristic cityscape of skyscrapers and sky transportation, resonating with President John F. Kennedy's call for Americans to claim space as the "new frontier" (see Fig. 3).[23] Man-made weather, as the imagery of advertisements conveyed, was part of a technocratic future in which more and more domains of life would be contained within a bubble of technological control, ensuring "optimum results" and "maximum efficiency."[24] Ventilation engineers regularly compared their sealed buildings to the automated space capsules promised for the near future, with their life-supporting artificial environments. Weather-making buildings "are fully air conditioned, just as space stations or a rocket carrying people to the moon will be,"[25] predicted a popular book on weather.

The connection between ventilation systems and the space age was, in fact, more than cold war imaginary. In 1959, with a new generation of engineers, ASHVE merged with the American Society of Refrigeration Engineers and became the American Society of Heating, Refrigerating, and Air-Conditioning Engineers (ASHRAE), moving its laboratory to the Institute of Environmental Research at Kansas State University in 1963.[26] ASHRAE's research money now came primarily from Department of Defense contracts. Its resources were devoted to the "study of the building of a system which will support life in a hostile environment such as outer space," as well as designs for nuclear and biological war shelters. Sealed spaces were artifacts of both the space race and the arms race.

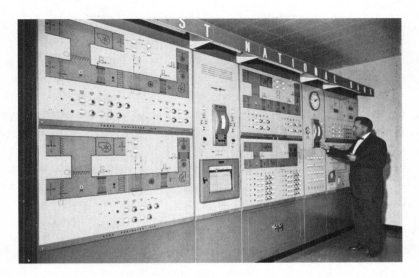

Figure 2. A central control console as celebrated on the cover of the *ASHRAE Journal*, November 1960. Reprinted by permission of ASHRAE.

Figure 3. Mid-century advertisements associated ventilation engineering with a future space age in which weather would be fully "mastered." Ventilation engineers were portrayed as dapper white men, dressed in professional suits and ties, whose technocratic prowess would automate the world. *ASHRAE Journal*, January 1959.

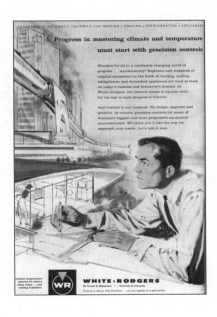

For ventilation engineers installing systems in the building boom of the 1950s, office buildings erected the interwar ventilation engineering assemblage. Strictly separating the inside from the outside with glass, they finally created a sealed box that could mechanically sustain the ventilation standards that had been developed in laboratories. They successfully delivered air-conditioned comfort, so how could one complain? Boxed up with unopenable yet sparkling windows, hidden from view in suspended ceilings, its thermostat safely out of the worker's reach, the office environment was under the firm control of technocratic engineers.

The postwar building-machine was a fetish not just of pedantic engineers but also of fashionable architects who designed corporate buildings. Some buildings even looked like machines. This well known modernist movement, called the "International Style" or "machine aesthetic," was famously influenced by European architects, such as Bauhaus architects Walter Gropius, Hannes Meyer, and Mies van der Rohe in Germany and Le Corbusier in France.[27] For Le Corbusier, who coined the term "machine for living," the building was a prosthetic—a technological extension of the human body—and should thus provide an ideal environment for human physiology. His normalized human, called the "Modulor," was linked to his plans for universalizable architecture through indoor climate: "Every nation builds houses for its own climate. At this time of international interpenetration of scientific techniques, I propose: one single building for all nations and climates, the house with respiration exact."[28]

With an imperialist rhetoric poised to capture the imagination of postwar corporations, the International Style made its way to America. With the rise of National Socialism and anti-Semitism in Germany, celebrity Bauhaus architects fled to Chicago, where they extolled the expression of function as an aesthetic. Exposing pipes and other building systems, using gleaming glass surfaces and durable concrete signified outwardly that buildings were indeed modern machines.[29] The New York– and Chicago-based architecture firm Skidmore, Owings, and Merrill (SOM) led the way in establishing the vernacular of American corporate modernism that would later devolve into the ubiquitous, square, glass buildings that dominated the information economy's architecture.[30] No longer simply built to shelter office work, office buildings were designed as a constituent part of the total corporate machine.[31] Prestigious office buildings designed by celebrity architects were constructed to facilitate physically the fashionable managerial interest in "rational," structuralist corporate systems.[32]

Rather than building up, this era sprawled out. When millions of white families migrated out of city centers to racially exclusive suburbs, corporate headquarters followed. Located in suburban isolation, the corporation spread vertically. Inside, it was segmented into departments according to function; when a new need arose, a new department was added to the corporate sprawl. Some departments, such as the mailroom, typewriting pool, and switchboard, were dedicated to the self-sufficiency of the entire machine. Others, like the newsstand, hairdresser, music room, library, shoeshine stand, or cafeteria provided amenities in suburban isolation. The general aesthetic favored was symmetrical, straight, sparse, tidy, and almost sterile. Interiors were illuminated with harsh florescent lighting, covered with polished hard vinyl flooring, and scrupulously clean. Ashtrays, nonetheless, perched next to electric pencil sharpeners, for smoking was a common and acceptable practice that did not tarnish the interior's clean sensibility.

Disparagingly dubbed the "Organization Man" in William Whyte's 1956 best-selling lament to the loss of individualism in a narrow world of affluence, the suburban corporate male manager expected to be rewarded for his conformity and loyalty with the security of a job for life.[33] The stereotype of the "Organization Man" was the organizational kin of the human norm ventilation engineers had charted. Organization Man's ability to never break a sweat in air-conditioned comfort was the prerogative in the 1950s and 1960s of the professional middle class.

The idealized sealed and sterilized world of corporate architecture encapsulated the isolationist mentality of the cold war and space age together with the narrow, racially exclusive bubble of white America's "Affluent Society."[34] Such suburban corporate headquarters were almost uniformly white, mixed gendered workplaces, with the exception of menial work like cleaning, maintenance, or shoeshining, all of which were occupations held as outside of and servile to the corporate family proper. The humanist notion of universal comfort implicit in ventilation standards was in practice an environmental marker of a historically particular, racialized class privilege. While one would certainly note the contrast between the summery or wintry outdoors and the ventilated interior, mechanically delivered comfort ideally allowed its beneficiaries to ignore the climate altogether. The environment of the office was distinguished precisely by being as imperceptible to its inhabitants as possible.

While for postwar social critics the sealed spaces of corporate America were a dangerous form of apathy and conformism, for corporate boosters they expressed a hopeful, technocratic futurism. Throughout the 1960s, the unquestioned goal of "space age" comfort was installed into office buildings according to the assemblage developed in the interwar period. Though the constituents of comfort were no longer examined, architects and engineers were engaged in figuring out how to practically deliver comfort to corporate environments. The phenomenon brought into being in the ASHVE labs was now materially ensconced in the corridors of corporate America.

The Flexible Machine and Naturalized Comfort

Imagine a real estate developer's plan for an office building at the dawn of the Reagan years. It will be constructed as an exterior shell, an empty box. Though made of glass, the windows will not open to save energy. The building will be surrounded by black asphalt parking lots, whose square footage precisely correlates to the square footage inside. A contractor will install the mass-produced HVAC units, one per section of the building, their modular boxes interrupting the flatness of the gravel roof. Inside, mechanical services will be hidden behind a white grid of suspended ceiling tiles that can easily be lifted so that wires and ducts can be moved. The building will be a shell whose insides can be altered. Because of this "flexibility," the building can be owned by one company and leased by another, with perhaps a third company contracted as building manager. The assemblage produced by ventilation engineering is now tied to a new logic: the construction of a building that can be leased for maximum profit.[35]

By the 1980s, ASHRAE represented a huge, billion-dollar industry. Contracting HVAC installation was a necessary part of real estate development. In the leasable office building, the sealed exterior surface and the openable interior surface combined to form a shell within which both the mechanical services and interior layouts could be altered depending on the whims of the renting corporation. The office building had become an empty box adjustable to different tenants.

In contrast to the mass-produced modular HVAC of the 1980s, the centralized environmental systems of the 1950s and 1960s were directly constructed into the architectural infrastructure. Years later, these systems were hard to access and usually too rigid to adapt to a company's reorganization. Office buildings of the 1970s and 1980s had to adjust physically to new information technologies, such as the video display terminal and the desktop computer, that required new kinds of wiring. Computers not only produced heat, they also required dry, dust-free environments, necessitating air conditioning for nonhuman reasons. The office design guru Robert Propst, who declared "change" as the new corporate master as early as 1968, identified the material construction of office buildings as one of the most significant obstacles to obeisance: "Our buildings, furnishings, and services . . . have to be revisualized and revitalized."[36] The modernist corporate machine was declared a sprawling mess too rigidly built to adapt to the ideology of change that characterized the "information age."[37] Bureaucracy was no longer a progressive project; it was a monolithic modernist monster to be slain. Even the modernist vision of a "machine for living," which rested on humanist principles, fell into disrepute as humanism itself was criticized by academics and famous modernist buildings were declared dysfunctional.[38] The successor office building was a rejection of static and centralized ventilation systems in favor of more "flexible" arrangements made of mass-produced parts that could be arranged to adapt to different markets. This much-applauded flexibility, however, was confined narrowly to the construction process. Office workers' access to the thermostat was rare, and thus so to was the "flexible" delivery of ventilation according to the desires of the individual. Ironically, the flexible system was intended to deliver a homogenous environment, typically the minimum mandated by ventilation codes as established during the interwar years.

By the 1980s, air conditioning itself was ubiquitous; even the masses could buy window models for their homes. Yet in the ventilation industry, active interrogation of the effects of ventilation on bodies had entirely ceased. Though part of a flexible construction process, mechanical services were unquestioningly expected to deliver a homogenous, comfortable, air-conditioned "comfort zone," now a naturalized, expected, and unremarkable part of the corporate environment. The profession of ventilation engineering was no longer the province of prestigious engineers affiliated with public health departments. Instead, ventilation was a self-evident and unglamorous part of the construction industry that was contracted out, often to small local firms, while the ventilation units themselves were assembled by rote as part of a mass-produced modular system, much like office furniture. Thus, unlike at mid century, even the installation of ventilation systems was rarely occasioned by feats of creative engineering. For the inhabitant, ventilation was black boxed: hidden from view in suspended ceilings, the thermostat out of reach. Even for the ventilation expert, HVAC was a black box about which few fundamental questions were asked. The idealistic concerns of modernist ventilation were not paid attention to—few people spoke any longer about · the effects of the indoor climate on bodies. Even though it was not spoken about, the assemblage of Man in a box was sedimented unquestioningly in buildings and building codes everywhere.

If anything was said about air conditioning, it related to the technology's very success and proliferation. The rapid spread of air conditioning in the 1960s and 1970s began to create summertime electricity shortages and blackouts. The tremendous suck on electricity caused by ubiquitous air conditioning, coupled with rising cost during the energy crisis of the early 1970s, resulted in a new market for energy-efficient construction. In 1974 ventilation standards were altered for the first time since 1938, but for reasons far removed from bodies.[39] The new standard emphasized energy efficiency, not worker efficiency or even comfort, reducing the minimum fresh air intake of buildings. The mechanical manufacture of comfort was materially inscribed in all office buildings, yet its relation to bodies disappeared from engineering research and construction.

The mechanical production of "comfort"—an odorless, sweatless, privileged environment—in office buildings was predicated on a relatively straightforward assemblage of building and body. The method of construction it gave rise to long outlived its founding rationale or discursive presence in the discipline. For the twentieth-century office managers who organized labor in these buildings, the comfortable office became the hallmark of a workplace that could painlessly extract labor from bodies. The success of the comfortable office, its seemingly naturalness, and the security it symbolized made it difficult for ventilation engineers, managers, occupational health experts, or even workers to imagine, let alone articulate, how such a space might inflict harm.

[2] **Crack open an office building** from the 1970s. Inside, the layouts of walls and windows, the distributions of desks, the pathways of paper, and the exertion of equipment formed tightly knit material and social assemblages for choreographing the labor of office workers. Both the building's shell and the population of furniture and machines in its interior were material arrangements designed to encourage what by the 1950s was called information work. The ducts, fans, and thermostats of the building-machine conspired with the files, keyboards, and cubicles of office work to actively shape the behavior and status of the people toiling within. As a physical arrangement of labor, the office interiors orchestrated technologies and architecture into a workplace that efficiently extracted labor from bodies, particularly the bodies of women clerical workers.

As the material manifestation of a new, peculiarly twentieth-century way of organizing work, these offices produced new rungs in the American class, race, and gender stratifications for workers to inhabit.[1] Harry Braverman, the well-known American socialist theorist, argued in his 1974 *Labor and Monopoly Capital* that "it is more accurate to see the clerical workers of the present monopoly capitalist era as virtually a new stratum. . . . Because if it is not, and if one ascribes to the millions of present-day clerical workers the 'middle class' or semi-managerial functions of that tiny and long-vanished clerical stratum of early capitalism, the result can only be a drastic misconception of modern society."[2] In the daily repetitions of office work, gender roles, in particular, were integral to the fashioning of new kinds of work for women at the bottom ranks of corporate America and at the same time the twentieth-century professional managerial middle class. As a relatively new domain and one of the largest to employ women, office buildings were important sites where gender was materialized, not just in relationship to masculine management, but also in relation to technologies, from filing cabinets to video display terminals (VDTS).

Office work, unlike ventilation engineering, had no single, simple, and distinctive assemblage that governed the status of laboring bodies within buildings. From clanking to buzzing, from bullpens to cubicles, from mechanical to digital, from steel to plastic, the components and materials that made up the built environment of office work changed dramatically over the twentieth century. Moreover, there was an ambiguity to the status of office workers, not only because notions of gender and race were shifting in American culture generally, but also because the way conflicts over what it meant to be an office worker were built into the air conditioners and paper trails of office buildings.

Power in offices, as in many other modern institutions, be they prisons or hospitals, was exercised in an abundance of small gestures, spatial boundaries, and paper trails—what the historian Michel Foucault called the "microphysics" of power—that governed subject positions, such as those of prisoner, patient, or secretary.[3] Yet the subject position of women office workers was not simply the formulaic outcome of the disciplinary strategies of management. On the one hand, what it meant to be an office worker was transformed by the people who daily inhabited the office building and intimately handled its technologies. On the other hand, offices were not coercive unities manipulating workers. Instead, they developed at the overlap of different managerial regimes instituted at different historical moments for assimilating humans into large corporate complexes.

"Information work" was a central site for investing in new affinities between the human and the machine. Discourses about the corporation as machine materially informed walls and workstations, managerial regimes and worker experiences. As fantasies and practicalities about what constituted the machinic were repeatedly reinvented over the course of the century, they were layered into the physicality of office work, not as a series of distinct phases, but rather more like sediment collecting in an aging formation. Within corporate spaces, office workers were not only raced, gendered, and classed, they were also *machined*. That is, the lowest ranks of office workers were apprehended as constituent parts of the corporate machine, subjected to modes of discipline based on changing machinic relations.

This chapter follows the history of the material culture of office work as a shifting assemblage of objects, architectural arrangements, and discourses interacting with bodies by virtue of ordering and controlling space, from Taylorized assembly lines to cybernetic networks. It argues that after a century of existence, tensions and fractures about the nature of the ideal worker and his or her efficient interface with technologies were built into the very pipes and paper trails of the office building. Office work depended on the way comfortable buildings built by ventilation engineers interpellated their inhabitants as privileged and the office as a site of respectability. The coexistence of ventilation systems and arrangements of office work fostered a fundamental tension within the material conditions of the office—the successful feminization of most kinds of nonmanagerial office work was tied to the emergence of a middle-class, comfortable ambiance that covered over class stratifications and eventually came to be an expectation associated with the job. Conditions that industrial workers routinely tolerated became absolutely unacceptable to the office worker, regardless of his or her rank. Yet, the bulk of office work was a lowly valued form of labor, gendered feminine and requiring the routinized manipulation of figures, text, and paper on light machinery. Thus, the built environment of office buildings was not the passive backdrop that ventilation engineers had intended; rather it actively choreographed laboring bodies.

This chapter traces in broad strokes the connections between technologies and bodies in twentieth-century offices and how women workers were placed by them, leaving for the next chapter how women office workers themselves apprehended these same material conditions.

Disciplining and Gendering Gesture

For greatest efficiency, it helps to set up your workstation like a production line. For example, organize paper, envelopes, forms, erasers, pens, pencils, and correcting materials so that a minimum of motion is necessary to obtain supplies and information.—Bernadine Branchaw et al., *Office Procedures for the Professional Secretary* (1984), 24

The modern office emerged in bits and pieces starting at the beginning of the twentieth century in the wake of the great industrial transformations of the previous century.[4] With the exceptions of banking and insurance, office work was at first a bookkeeping addendum peripheral to the main manufacturing concern of most companies. In the early twentieth century, an emergent "progressive," college-educated, male, managerial class brought "scientific management" and the organizational principles of Fredrick Taylor to industries; with Taylorism the office began to outstrip the shop floor as the locus for managerial control of industrial labor.[5] Scientific management evolved as a set of technologies—mechanical, informational, and sociological—for ordering and controlling large organizations, such as factories, government bureaucracies, railroad companies, and insurance firms. In their application of "scientific" accounting methods, managers used time cards to track costs in terms of time, labor, and materials. The data collected on these time cards were calculated using machines such as the comptometer and the tabulator; this information was then subjected to efficiency analyses and systematically filed. Rationalization meant order through calculability; stop watches, recording devices, time cards, accounting methods, and calculating machines translated work into numbers that provided a powerful tool for controlling the labor process.

The tasks of generating and tracking this information spawned innumerable mechanical devices. The influential Computing Tabulating Recording Company, for example, was founded in 1911 and became better known under its later name, the International Business Machines Corporation (IBM).[6] Someone had to spend the tedious hours pushing small buttons, punching precise holes, and turning finicky cranks on these new technologies, so with each machine came a new job. Job titles often represented workers as if they had seamlessly joined the technology they operated: stenographer, comptometer, switch, addressographer, tabulator, typewriter, and keypuncher.[7] Broadly speaking, two new categories of workers were created through scientific management: the gendered male manager, either college-educated or promoted from a clerk position, and the gendered female office worker who did the manual labor of operating office machinery (see Figs. 4 and 5).

In the late nineteenth century, "ladies" began to be hired as office workers, introducing a strong discourse of gender into the office. By the 1930s, young European-American women, or "girls," from both working- and middle-class backgrounds were hired to run routinized office machinery, turning office work into a highly feminized occupation associated with machines designed to require a stereotyped nimble feminine

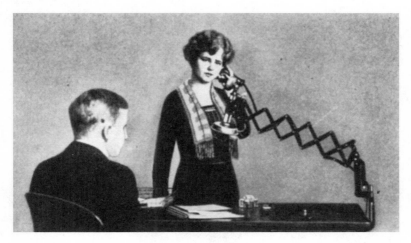

Figure 4. The gendered division of labor in the scientifically managed office was explicit in guidebooks of the early twentieth century. In this 1926 illustration from William Leffingwell's *Office Appliance Manual*, an "easily and instantly adjustable" telephone bracket juxtaposes attention to efficiency at the gestural level and the gender normalization of who appropriately operates the telephone. The bracket economizes the female worker's labor, which in turn shields the male manager from operating light machinery. Leffingwell, *Office Appliance Manual*.

touch. White women quickly came to predominate in office buildings numerically, populating the lowest rungs of the office hierarchy, creating a so-called "pink-collar" class amid white-collar work. Typewriter and stenography work was exemplary of this trend. While in 1900 women accounted for 76.7 percent of 112,699 workers, by 1930 women were 95.6 percent of 811,200 workers.[8] This new class of office workers was overwhelmingly European American. Racial discrimination and institutionalized segregation made it extremely rare for an African-American or Asian-American woman, no matter how well trained, to get an office job at a white-owned company.[9] Even for European-American women, there were only a few kinds of occupations open to them. Even newspaper advertisements for office job openings were explicitly categorized by race and sex well into the 1960s. White, working-class women were attracted to office over factory work because of its safety and cleanliness, its atmosphere of middle-class respectability, and even its glamour coded through dress, grooming, decor, and manners. Office work was

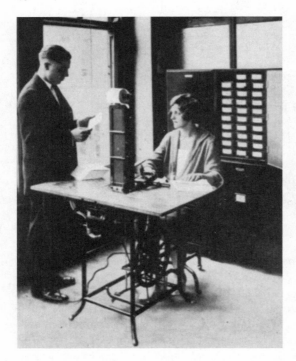

Figure 5. This photograph of the ideal setup of an addressing machine and its corresponding file system exemplifies the typical representation of gender in scientific management. The male manager, in a suit, is standing reading out a command; the female worker, with short hair and middle-class dress, is sitting operating light machinery. Leffingwell used this particular illustration to demonstrate "what little space is required." Leffingwell, *Office Appliance Manual.*

desirable work, and young white women flocked to be typewriters or stenographers, pushing the boundaries of company dress regulations with their fashionable attire. A fantasy of romance also shaped the mixed-sex workplace of the office, in which stylish, single young women worked for bachelor managers.

Educated, middle-class women were also attracted to office work. For them it was one of the few socially sanctioned opportunities to earn a wage; office work helped women to bring needed income to their birth families, while maintaining their middle-class respectability. The middle-class presentation of the office also developed conversely; as women were increasingly present, male workers modified their behavior, curbing, for example, their swearing and spitting. "Ladies"—always white—were held as a civilizing force in the office, and thus had to exhibit the moral qualities of civilization. Yet for women, unlike male clerks, the "marriage bar" and sex discrimination ensured that there was little expectation of promotion; before the Second World War it was commonplace for women to quit when they married.

The organization of the early-twentieth-century office, moreover, not only relied on sex-segregated and raced divisions of labor, it also shaped what kind of work was considered appropriate to women. The influential manual *Office Management* (1927) by William Leffingwell, which brought Taylorism to office work, advised that a woman was preferred for certain kinds of labor "for she is not averse to doing minor tasks, work involving the handling of petty details, which would irk and irritate ambitious young men."[10] Office buildings, thus, had become an important cultural site at mid century where white women from both middle-class and working-class backgrounds daily handled new technologies designed especially for their allegedly "nimble fingers," thereby shaping the very definition of "women's work."

Since the office sprang from the scientific management of industrial work, it is not surprising that the disciples of Taylor quickly rationalized the office as well.[11] Leffingwell was the foremost of these disciples and even designed office furniture to rouse women to even greater heights of productivity (see Fig. 6). As in the factory, scientific management saw the worker's movements and the machine she operated as a unit that could be disassembled into standardizable parts. Any individual task was broken down into constituent gestures, and the time it took to complete each of these motions was then measured. The pushing, punching, and handle turning required by office machinery was particularly amenable to the application of Taylorism.

The lowest status workers, most vulnerable to the machined disciplining of their gestures, were physically restricted to their desks, which were arranged in symmetrical rows within a room often called the "bullpen." The rows of workstations facing forward in a large common room allowed workers to be scrutinized by the constant gaze of a supervisor, who might be stationed on a raised platform at the front like a schoolteacher. The female-populated bullpen was physically separated from the work of male management by walls and soundproofing.[12] Within a

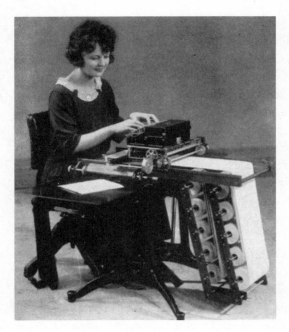

Figure 6. Illustrations of office machinery were conventionally portrayed with a person as operator, most typically a young woman. This photograph, described as an illustration of a noncomputing biller, is typical for the way it uses a female model but does not explicitly comment on her presence, thereby eliding her with the machine she operates. Operators are posed as if playing a piano, in a way that underlines the gendering of a kind of physical nimbleness. Note the figure's dress, short hair, and stiff posture. From Leffingwell, *Office Appliance Manual*.

bullpen, women could work all day on a single machine, or even a single task on a machine, and were often paid by piecework, making it very similar to the factory floor. With its successive small movements and long hours sitting in one place, this labor required that women workers not only to be skilled with their fingers, likened in advertisements to the middle-class skill of piano playing, but also to subject their bodies to the routinization of rationalized machinery. The early-twentieth-century office-as-factory, then, materialized women as gendered, raced, and machined subjects integrated as mechanical components of a gesturally controlled assembly line. Standardized motion could be thought of as interchangeable parts from which office managers could assemble their offices. Office work for most women was manual, not mental work— hand, not head work. By the Second World War, office work required highly disciplined female bodies that could efficiently perform small repetitive gestures and at the same time comply with middle-class standards of dress and comportment.

Total Worlds and Patriarchal Families

Each office within the skyscraper is a segment of the enormous file, a part of the symbol factory that produces ten billion slips of paper that gear modern society into its daily shape.—C. Wright Mills, *White Collar* (1953), 189

In the economic and construction boom that followed the Second World War, the technologies that organized the modern office, which had been haphazardly introduced, became solidified into elaborate paper factories. The mid-century construction of modern, air-conditioned office buildings blessed the workers within with technological luxury and physical comfort. The sealed, streamlined, and, later, space-age offices, and the comfortable, odorless environment allowed the lowest typist and the highest managers to rub elbows in a common space. The sparkling glass-and-steel architecture of mid-century office buildings was glamorously outfitted by the modernist furniture of industrial designers such as Charles and Ray Eames, George Nelson, Florence Knoll, and Harry Bertoia. The ambiance represented office work as pleasant, even luxurious, and as a progressive site of "tomorrow's world."

The "symbol factory" residing in sparkling downtown skyscrapers and suburban headquarters was not only a showplace for modern design, it also housed corporations that fashioned themselves as "total worlds" in which all of a company's needs, from social occasions for its staff to research and development departments, were part of a large, self-sustained corporation. The new problem of managing large-scale payrolls and billing, as well as forecasting and marketing, required new methods for administrating office labor with "totally integrated management systems" that drew from operations systems management developed during the war.[13] Before the late 1950s, managers spoke of "facts," not "information." Calling office work "information work" invoked the scientificity of the exciting new field of information theory, as well as the growing application of punch-card computers to administrative tasks. "Systems men" of the newly founded Systems and Procedures Association, chartered in 1947, promoted the use of standardized forms and the redesign of clerical procedures as well as the writing of corporate technical manuals. Similar to the central control console of ventilation engineering, which controlled a building's services, systems men strove to integrate all functions into a single management system facilitated by computing, a system that automated managers as much as clerical workers.[14]

Inside the office buildings that systems men sought to manage, labor was segmented by task and status according to a finely gradated and gendered hierarchy that divided work into smaller and smaller units to form a pyramidal organization called "functional specialization." In this pyramid, the smaller the unit of work one was responsible for, the lower one's rank in the corporate hierarchy.[15] Within the hive of individual offices that marked territory within the corporation, furniture, style, and office size denoted which rung on the corporate ladder a worker stood on.[16] Office furniture manufacturers, such as Herman Miller, Steelcase, and Knoll, began specializing in elaborate, clean-lined, mass-produced steel and plywood furniture systems that could signal status in the office hierarchy by the color, size, and style of furniture and equipment. The Union Carbide Building, for example, designed by the architectural firm Skidmore, Owings, and Merrill, was constructed between 1955 and 1960 in downtown Manhattan. This fifty-two-story tower of steel-framed, gray-tinted glass took the systemization of office furniture to the extreme of assigning each job category its own color and style of pen, ashtray, and coffee cup (see Fig. 7).[17] Such furniture systems worked not only to demarcate status, but also as surveillance mechanisms—workers could easily interpret each other's status and could just as easily recognize its infringement.

In the words of Herman Miller's George Nelson, the design of furniture "communicated" something to its user, interpolating him or her into a specific status in the hierarchy. The executive office was typically set apart as an elaborate suite with a large imposing wooden desk, expensive art hanging on the wall, an elegant leather armchair, and a bar for refreshments, resembling the domestic space of an elite living room. In the rest of the office, the aesthetic was more austere and geometrical,

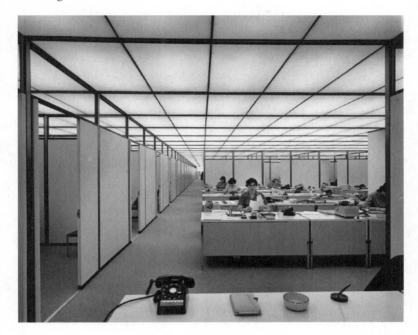

Figure 7. Interior of the Union Carbide headquarters in New York City, designed by the architectural firm of Skidmore, Owings, and Merrill in 1960. The headquarters was designed as a total system, down to the pens, ashtray, and address file in the foreground. Women who worked as secretaries were situated in a central space adjacent to the private offices of the men whom they served. Note the straight lines, symmetry, and functional aesthetic. Photograph by Ezra Stoler. © Esto.

even sterile. The managerial class of white men, each with his own purposeful private office with wooden L-shaped desk and comfortable chair, oversaw a specific function or department. The secretary, in contrast, sat in a simple armless chair behind a metal and plywood desk on which perched a variety of light machinery, from telephone to typewriter to pencil sharpener. Her wall-less or glass-walled office was typically located in front of the office of the man whom she served. From nine to five, though in close proximity, men and women inhabited very different physical spaces and worked with quite different technologies.

Within the total office system, the trope of the heterosexual and patriarchal family remained crucial to organizing the divisions of labor within a mixed-sex workplace, as well as the work roles available to women, ranging from wife to girl.[18] Women's office work was divided between those women who were front-office workers, such as secretaries, assigned to work for one man and back-office workers assigned to specific machines. Secretarial work required a host of specialized and "feminine" skills that were more difficult to mechanize and thus more closely matched the ideals of white-collar work. Secretaries were an integral part of the white-collar corporate family, sometimes referred to as the "second wives" of the men they served. They were required to fetch coffee, buy Christmas gifts, greet visitors, and dial the phone for their bosses in a system sociologist Barbara Garrison labeled as "office monogamy."[19]

The relationship between a male manager and his personal secretary paralleled the conservative gender division of work that predominated in the professional white middle class of the 1950s and 1960s. In this emerging class, both sexes might be college educated, but only the husbands typically had careers. Once married, house servants of previous decades were replaced by the laboring wife and her washing machine in a gender ideology that placed middle-class women as the servants of their spouses and children, creating a gigantic gap in the value of the labor done by the two sexes in a middle-class marriage.[20] At mid century, it was common for women to do the manual labor for male managers both at home and at work.

The personal secretary's intimate relationship with management, the valuing of middle-class social skills and dress, and her varied tasks stood in stark contrast to the work of the "girls" operating office machinery in typing pools or at switchboards. Only the more prestigious job of the well-dressed secretary was visible to management. Routinized office work, as with the earlier bullpen, was kept out of management's sight in backrooms and basements, in the same way that the building's pipes, ducts, and wires were hidden behind suspended ceilings and walls. Even for these workers, the middle-class, air-conditioned environment, with amenities such as restrooms, locker rooms, and lunchrooms, was crucial to their work and self-identity. As African-American women agitated to be hired into the ranks of office workers as part of the civil rights movement, Euro-American women resisted, invoking the exclusiveness of their racialized status as "ladies." For companies, investing low-ranking jobs with a middle-class ambiance could protect against pressure to desegregate.[21]

Within this exclusive architectural and social matrix, a new group of office technologies began to replace the hefty metal machines powered by human muscle. The clacking of mechanical keys was replaced by the electric buzz of the IBM Selectric typewriter, introduced in 1961. Durable concrete, wood, and steel were replaced by a growing wave of synthetic material—such as Formica, fiberglass, and polyurethane. "Mistake Out," later to become Liquid Paper, began to be sold in 1956. In 1959 Xerox unveiled its first xerographic automatic office copier, which soon became a fixture in every office. By 1965 a third generation of computers with integrated circuits and standardized business programs, though still bulky and slow, was being introduced into office work.[22] From plastic telephone cases to molded fiberglass chairs to asbestos ceiling tiles, the materials and substances housed in the sealed corporate world were changing.[23]

Nodes in the Cybernetic Network

In the past, it was comforting to be part of stable, permanent organizations. Change, with its newness and novelty, was limited to the role of upgrading or improving existing forms. History has taught us to accept the straight line of evolution. We are disturbed by the revolutionary effect of exponential change rates. Undeniably, we are already deeply involved with a new state of reality, a new iron mistress, the exponential change in the rate of change. The office in its relationship to the organization it serves must now obey the dynamic new factors this imposes.—Robert Propst, *The Office: A Facility Based on Change* (1968), 24

In 1968 Robert Propst, an industrial designer at Herman Miller, published a manifesto that declared "change" to be the new master of office organization. The successor office, he declared, rejected static, geometric, and functionalist arrangements in favor of a "flexible" or "open system" that could adapt to changing technologies and markets. This new type of changeable arrangement was initially inspired by the cybernetic approach to systems, pioneered and popularized by Norbert Wiener from the 1940s through the 1960s, but which came to the office by way of Germany.[24] In 1968, the Quickborner Team, made up of brothers Eberhard and Wolfgang Schnelle, designed a radically new form of office organization called *office landscaping* or *open planning*.[25] As with

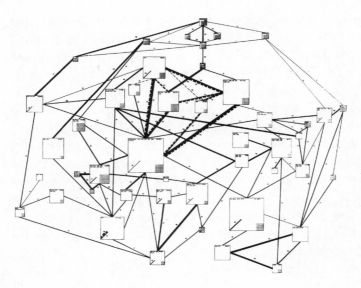

Figure 8. Quickborner Team diagram of communication flow (lines) between work groups (represented by boxes) from which they purportedly
planned the layout of an open plan office.

Wiener's cybernetic weapons guidance mechanism, the open plan was
designed to reduce error and increase efficiency by constantly adjusting
the office apparatus.[26]

According to the Quickborner plan, offices should be organized, not by
hierarchy or department, but through the democratic circulation of information. Of the sixty-eight Quickborner Team rules for office landscaping,
the most important was "An office is a center for communication information processing. Work relationships are not to be understood in terms
of administrative departmental organization, nor in terms of rank and
status, but only as matters of communication flow."[27] The Quickborner
Team logged an office's traffic of communication—on paper, by face-to-
face conversation, and by telephone—using surveys and then turned the
results into charts of the flow of communication between workers (see
Fig. 8). The confusing matrix of connecting lines in such charts invoked
electrical circuit diagrams, signaling to the viewer that open-plan offices
were not symmetrical hierarchies but instead were engineered according
to the dictates of a communication flow that necessarily violated class.
The hives of individual offices for management typical of modernism

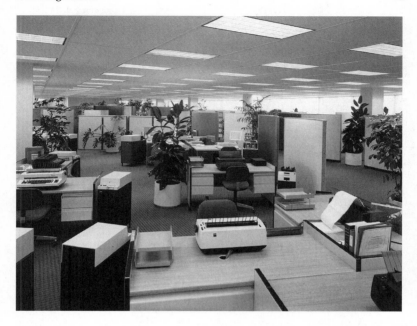

Figure 9. Open plan office in the Montgomery Ward Headquarters, Chicago, October 1973. In this interior a Steelcase 900 furniture system was arranged without symmetry, potted plants invoked the sense of "office landscaping," and wall-to-wall carpeting and textiled partitions helped to muffle noise. Photographed by Hedrich Blessing, HB-38733. Courtesy of the Chicago Historical Society.

were replaced with an unrestricted, environmentally uniform open space where, ideally, the adjustable plastic modular furniture of all workers—from the highest executive to the lowest clerical worker—could be arranged to maximize the efficiency of this flow. Efficiency of communication, not hierarchy or aesthetics, was the single valid reason for placing workers near to or far from one another, since individual workers were seen as nodes in a communication network. To muffle the noise created by so many people in a large open space, all open-plan offices replaced hard-surfaced floors with plush carpets and lined the walls with synthetic textiles. Office *landscaping*, moreover, called for potted plants and cheerful colors to maintain the sense that the office was a pleasant and comfortable environment (see Fig. 9).

In 1967, DuPont became the first company in the United States to

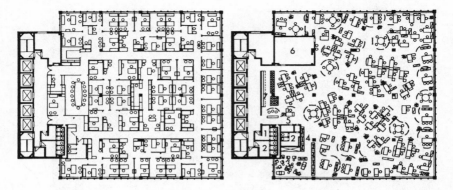

Figure 10. A conventional office floor plan with symmetrically arranged individual offices is compared with an open floor plan in a 1967 trial arrangement at DuPont by the Quickborner Team. This was the first open plan office in America. From "Burolandschaft U.S.A," *Progressive Architecture*, May 1968.

install an open-plan test site (diagrammed in Fig. 10). The Quickborner Team's before-and-after diagram of this test site circulated widely in architectural circles. It served as a visual exemplar of how old-fashioned symmetrical office space was being replaced by a seemingly random arrangement of furniture that was shocking to the corporate aesthetic of status and order. Eastman Kodak, Corning Glass, Ford Motor, Aetna, and IBM soon followed Dupont. In America, however, the strict rule-bound Quickborner Team plan was quickly refashioned into a watered-down American-style open plan. Executives and high-level managers retained their private offices and open planning was restricted to front office workers and lower-level management positions, while the back office remained separate and out of sight. In America, the open-plan office was popularized by Herman Miller under the guidance of industrial designers George Nelson and Robert Propst. Propst's widely used "Action Office," a steel, plywood, and laminate modular furniture "system," was the precursor to the cubicle. Instead of emphasizing open spaces, the Action Office replaced solid walls with light and bright movable partitions that contained adjustable furniture, lighting, and storage. Propst used time-lapse photography to study the habits of ordinary office workers at their desks and interviewed "high performance" workers like Polaroid inventor Edwin Land, anthropologist Margaret Mead, and comedian Steve Allen. Propst's open-plan office resulted not from a cybernetic analysis of information flow but from his belief that desk work needed to be made more efficient and the ideological shift toward flexibility instantiated in accordance with the more general restructuring of corporations that began in the late 1960s.[28]

Within this restructuring, finely gradated pyramid hierarchies located in a single building were replaced with a new organization of concentric circles in which the core was the most stable and the farther rings were attached by increasingly contingent types of employment.[29] The core was made up of absentee stockholders who owned the company, a small core of top executives with extremely high salaries and private suites, and a stable high-level managerial class, educated at business schools, who enjoyed job security. The largest group of employees—a middle ring of bureaucrats, middle managers, and administrative assistants (who used to be called secretaries)—had less security and more "flexibility." Their exact function and number varied according to demand. The farthest ring consisted of part-time, temporary, customer service, and back-office workers who increasingly worked on VDTs. These workers moved from the basement or back office to an "administrative center" often located in a separate building and only attached to the corporation by contract. As computer networks became less encumbered with the physical limitations of proximity through telecommunications, back-office work could be sent to distant locations, or "outsourced."[30]

By the 1980s, tasks such as customer service, order taking, and data entry were outsourced to other firms in economically cheaper peripheral locations, sometimes even overseas, where workers could be hired for low pay. These new information workers labored in front of the green glow of electronically surveilled video monitors. Out of sight and off-site, women of color increasingly occupied such low-visibility, outsourced positions. Even in these information work environments, however, air-conditioning, carpeting, and "professional" attire signaled to women that they were not the comrades of women working on the factory floor. Nor was outsourced data processing work linked to the labor of assembling computing and electronic technologies, work also performed by young women working in a different node of the vast currents of information in the global economy. The feminist critic Rachel Grossman developed the vivid concept of "women in the integrated circuit" in 1980 to connect the lives of women subsisting, and resisting, within the multiple global manifestations of the information economy, from offices to the electronic assembly lines of Southeast Asia and New Mexico.[31] For management, assembly-line work, vulnerable to the whims of contracting in the global economy, stood outside the concentric circles of the office proper. So did the labor in call centers and data-processing services operated by contractors. Moreover, within American office buildings themselves was another invisible group working in the integrated circuit: women and men of color or new immigrants who, before the sun rose, maintained the pleasant appearance of the office using a multitude of "industrial strength" detergents and disinfectants. Thus, the "reengineering" of office work in the 1970s and 1980s involved a reconfiguration of what jobs were considered inside the boundaries of corporate office work and which were considered outside.

The cybernetic ideal of office interiors as forming an efficient and adaptive integrated circuit was rarely materialized beyond the initial experiments in the late 1960s. Even those companies that initially organized their offices according to communication-flow studies did not follow these guidelines in subsequent adaptations. The open office did not become widespread because it arranged communication efficiently. Despite democratizing ideals of interrank communication, the open plan quickly prospered because it allowed companies to squeeze larger numbers of workers into smaller spaces.[32] The modular furniture systems were replaced with a warren of chipboard and synthetic textile cubicles. In the past, women in the typing pool worked in a common space that allowed for some socializing. With cubicles, the view of colleagues was cut off. Although they occupied a common space, workers found themselves isolated, as one woman described: "Now they have a new set-up, called the 'open office' where I work. . . . There are panels 6 feet high around all the operators. We're divided into work groups of 4 to 6, with a supervisor for each group. In many cases, we don't see another person all day except for a 10-minute coffee break and lunch time. All we see is the walls around us and sometimes the supervisors. The isolation is terrible."[33]

Cubicle systems—nicknamed "veal fattening pens" in Douglas Copeland's acute novel of late-twentieth-century life, Generation X—were made of plastic or particle-board walls, lined with synthetic textiles, that came in a variety of colors and sizes.[34] The square footage of a cubicle was determined by rank. The following assignments were typical of

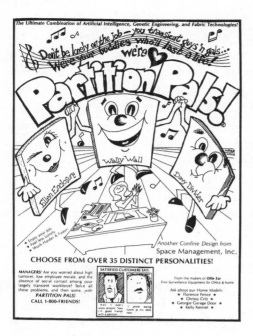

Figure 11. A cartoon from the San Francisco zine *Processed World* (1981), which was dedicated to critiquing information work as an element of late capitalism. This cartoon contrasted the "humanizing" marketing of office furniture with the isolation it could produce. Courtesy of *Processed World*, www.processedworld.com.

office design manuals: manager, 154 square feet; secretary, 64 square feet; data retrieval worker, 56 square feet; data entry worker, 48 square feet; and typist, 41 square feet.[35] The height of the cubicle could also vary according to worker status.

Progressive companies sometimes allowed workers to pick the color of their cubicles under a philosophy called "participatory design."[36] The Union Carbide headquarters built in 1987, in dramatic contrast to the color hierarchy system of its headquarters built in the 1950s, allowed each worker to pick a color and model from a selection of thirteen desks, fifteen chairs, one hundred fabric swatches, six credenzas, ten telephone colors, and even six different in and out baskets.[37] Participatory design was promoted as a boon to productivity: "Uninspiring work can be tolerated if employees have the right to exercise influence over other areas of their work lives."[38] With participatory design, workers were provided with an illusory sense of control over their workplaces by allowing them to participate in trivial decisions, distracting them from analyzing the way power operated in the office apparatus (this dynamic is satirized in the cartoon shown in Fig. 11).

The success of participatory design at AT&T was summarized by one

designer as "more people . . . put in less space at lower first cost and lower
long-term cost, with an increase in environmental satisfaction."[39] In this
way, participatory design drew on a tradition of "human relations" management responsible for the famous Hawthorne experiment, conducted
at the Western Electric Company between 1924 and 1933 by Elton Mayo
and his colleagues at the Harvard Business School.[40] These studies began
with an investigation into the effect of illumination on industrial worker
productivity, finding that productivity increased whether lighting levels
were increased or decreased. Similar results came from an experiment
with six women working in a relay assembly test room. While this experiment found that the women's productivity increased as the work conditions were improved by the researchers through breaks, shorter hours,
and better lighting, it also found that productivity continued to increase
after all these special improvements were removed. What came to be
called the "Hawthorne Effect" in social science research was how the
attention of the researchers overwhelmed the effects of changes to the
work environment.

The Hawthorne experiments were widely taken by managers as evidence that workers' need for recognition and a sense of belonging was
more important to them than the physical environment of the workplace. For managers, the experiments also showed that workers' complaints revealed not so much a real problem in the workplace as the
employees' dissatisfaction with their status and social position. Participatory design, like the Hawthorne experiments, was thought to increase
productivity by giving workers a sense that management was attentive to
their needs, while at the same time relieving management of making
substantive material or social changes to the workplace environment.

As more and more offices became labyrinths of cubicles, the interest
in communication flow that characterized the early open plan did not
entirely disappear; instead it morphed into a new form that harkened
back to the scientific management regimes of the 1930s. With the use of
VDTs and later of desktop computers in the early 1980s, the data input of
each worker could be precisely and continually recorded without requiring face-to-face interaction, allowing managers to monitor the efficiency
of workers digitally, to a degree impossible with Taylorist time-motion
studies.[41] Unlike Taylorism, electronic monitoring was not used to study
body motion and posture (now part of the field of ergonomics that was
incorporated into furniture design); rather, it concentrated on creating

statistics on error, speed, idle time, and seconds per customer—effectively turning computer work into highly regimented piecework. The sociologist Shoshana Zuboff dubbed this method of worker control "the information panopticon."[42] While advertisers coded the computer as masculine, figures of data entry inevitably displayed a woman's hands.[43] With the continued feminization of data entry, women remained symbolically absorbed as part of the machine itself. The person and the machine were persistently conflated in job titles—then "typewriter," now "data processor"—represented as mere conduits in a larger system.

In 1970, office work in the United States employed 13.7 million clerical workers; 74.6 percent of whom were women.[44] Although most clerical workers were still white at this time, after the Civil Rights Act of 1963, African-American and other women of color made significant inroads into clerical work, especially in government bureaucracy.[45] In 1960, only 8 percent of black women workers were employed as clericals; in 1980, by contrast, clerical work accounted for 29 percent of black women's employment and 36.5 percent of white women's.[46] Middle management positions also had become increasingly open to educated white middle-class women, blurring the former distinction between male manager and female underling. Feminized clerical work had also become more proletarianized relative to the variety of occupations white middle-class women now pursued. This trend was demonstrated both in the insecurity of the employment and in women's pay: beginning in 1970 the median salary of clerical workers was lower than that of every type of blue-collar work.[47] In the "cybernetic office," some office workers began to see themselves as a new class of laborers aligned with rather than different from factory workers. Karen Nussbaum, a founder of 9to5, the National Organization of Women Office Workers, described this new working class: "No longer is the typical American worker a man in a hard hat. The typical worker is a woman at a typewriter or, rather, a keyboard."[48]

The insecurity that plagued the so-called flexible workplace, the low wages back-office workers were paid, the shifting locations of information work in the global economy, and the upward mobility of white middle-class women into management juxtaposed against continued sex-segregation of now racially diverse clerical work all helped to shatter the modernist pretense of happy and loyal "girls" within a corporate family. Yet, even the lowliest data processing took place in a carpeted, clean, and air-conditioned space, necessitated as much by the environmental needs of computers as the maintenance of a middle-class ambiance. By the 1970s, women office workers were poised to respond to the hail of a newly reconfigured feminism, which would allow them to rematerialize the terms of the office.

Building Discipline and Comfort

Office work over the course of the twentieth century was characterized by a fundamental tension: a form of physical labor requiring the gendering and machining of bodies, office work also took place in a comfortable and safe environment engineered to be unsensed and designed for prestige. The middle-class gendering of office work that was built into its very walls was fundamental to the covering over of class stratifications that were built into its very machines. Ventilation engineering and office work, which developed as distinct domains for materially arranging buildings and bodies, nonetheless shared notions of efficiency and machinery, from Taylorized assembly lines to centralized systems and flexible cybernetic networks. The building environment designed by ventilation engineers worked closely together with the interior layout organized by management to compose the everyday manifestation of information work. While these two manifestations of office buildings often worked together and administered bodies similarly (e.g., they both materialized bodies as machines), they also conflicted. This conflict could at times be an important aspect of the extraction of labor from bodies: disciplining via, not despite, comfort.

Notwithstanding the continuity of this paradox over the century, office work itself underwent significant changes in the types of technologies, building materials, and management ideologies through which workers were interpellated. Nonetheless, offices continued to be segregated by sex, with labor strictly gendered. Women and men not only worked in different areas, they also handled different technologies. Thus, the effects of office work on bodies were also gendered. The comfortable built environment and the middle-class trappings made it difficult for workers, managers, or occupational health experts to articulate how office work was exploitative, or how it might inflict itself on bodies. When women voiced their first complaints about the health effects of office work, it was easy to dismiss them as trivial.

Feminism, Surveys, and Toxic Details

Office workers are not falling off tall buildings, emerging at 5pm covered with soot, or getting their hands caught in dangerous machines. But as an understanding of chemical and psychological hazards has increased, we have learned that office workers are exposed to severe dangers, all the more severe because they are often invisible and unrecognized.—Ellen Cassedy, 9to5, 1979

[3] **Black lung, brown lung,** silicosis, asbestosis, radiation poisoning —these are the kinds of diseases that spring to mind when we think of occupational health in twentieth-century America.[1] Compared to the mechanical and chemical hazards of industrial work that led to loss of limb and life, the carpeted, air-conditioned, clean interiors of late-capitalist office work appeared benign refuges from occupational disease and explicit exploitation. For ventilation engineers and corporate managers, as I argued in chapters 1 and 2, office buildings were materially arranged as efficient and even comfortable places for the extraction of labor. Both of these disciplines were undergirded by assemblages that gendered workers into universalized bodies amenable to mechanical control. However, the actual typists, secretaries, and data processors inhabiting offices were not fully captured by this portrait; in their daily lives as office workers they might struggle to dress appropriately, feel harassed by their boss, find an office machine clumsy, or read novels at breaks. While the office, relative to the factory, was indeed comfortable and safe, those attributes only partially captured the corporeal experience of office work. As a feminized labor force, moreover, office workers in the 1970s were poised to answer the hail of a resurgent feminism that disrupted the pacified gender roles the office relied on, summoning women as critical embodied registers of the effects of patriarchy.[2]

How did the women office workers' movement rematerialize the effects of office work when office buildings were designed to supply a neutral, hence comfortable, environment? Rematerialization was not simply in the negative, a "saying no" to the coercion of the office; nor was it a liberation or escape from office work. Rematerialization involved the production of an alternative way of assembling office work and bodies together that allowed workers to detect and articulate a previously unmarked oppression that required intervention. The built environment of the office was not just an external, a priori thing that workers simply responded to, were effected by, or understood more or less accurately. Instead, women office workers were part of the office and could instigate new means of inhabiting it, thus making the office a different kind of place. Forming a movement, office workers brought together vernacular technoscience and feminist practices that imbued office work with some characteristics and not others. Through their social and technical assemblage, the office became composed of an oppressive tide of small details, what one could call the microphysics of office work.[3] Instead of a machine for extracting efficiency in a pleasant environment, the office was rematerialized as a site of oppression and pathology. In the following pages, I argue that materializations from below—by office workers who were feminists and labor activists—were made possible by a technoscientific assemblage requiring as much skill with bodies, language, and artifacts as the highest technoscientific materializations.[4] Their rendering of office work uneasily coexisted with, rather than negated, the comfortable climate and efficient spatial arrangements that made up the material culture of office buildings.

Office workers in the 1970s had no specific disease for doctors to diagnose nor acute chemical exposure for investigators to measure. Office workers instead claimed that they experienced a multitude of minor corporeal distresses in myriad and seemingly innocuous circumstances. If occupational illness was generated by office work, the "nature" of that illness contravened conventional understandings of occupational disease. At the beginning of the twentieth century, the "nature" of occupational health had been formulated in terms of industrial accidents identifiable in time and place. Accidents and their compensation were codified in schedules: lose an arm, receive X amount of money.[5] In the 1930s workers' compensation boards expanded their compass by adding select industrial diseases to schedules. Newly established industrial hygiene laboratories identified occupational diseases in terms amenable to the logic of industrial accidents: as a predictable disease, such as lead poisoning, that an acute exposure to a specific chemical caused. Such occupational diseases could be specified and compensated as predictable and regular results of exposures that could be pinpointed.[6] Thus scientists developed technologies such as blood tests, X-rays, air samplers, and exposure chambers to render perceptible specific and predictable causal pathways between an identified workplace exposure and its corresponding physiological expression.[7] Enshrined in investigation protocols, juridical precedents, and workers' compensation rules, the use of such technologies and the formulation of specific causality became necessary to prove the very existence of occupational illness. In this specific sense, however, there was no "disease" associated with office work. If occupational illness was to be associated with office work, its nature defied causal specificity and the search for discrete disease entities. Thus, the women office workers' movement had to offer an alternative version of how workplaces might affect bodies.

The identification of modern occupational health problems—from black lung to sick building syndrome (sbs)—has more often been the result of grassroots struggle than medical detective work. Most incidents of occupational illness, community chemical exposures, and cancer clusters in the twentieth-century United States would not have become recognized without the vernacular technoscientific practices of workers and lay people, often called "popular epidemiology."[8] The efforts of the women office workers' movement of the 1970s and 1980s to name and apprehend occupational health problems in the office is an example. Activists and advocacy groups such as 9to5, the National Organization of Women Office Workers, drew on feminist and scientific methods to materialize the corporeal effects of office work, maintaining that, despite appearances, office work generated dispersed, insidious, and gendered forms of oppression that were individually negligible, but that were nonetheless rendered legible as a collectivity. Instead of housing specific, chemically induced industrial diseases, office hazards were *nonspecific*, subtle assaults caused by seemingly banal technologies and trivialized work practices.

Feminism in the Office

The women's liberation movement appears to be on the threshold of a second phase—when feminist consciousness reaches beyond white, middle-class women . . . [A] clear sign of the new awareness felt by the so-called typical woman is the way office workers are asserting themselves. There is nothing quite so typical as a woman who is a secretary, typist, clerk, or keypunch operator.—Margie Albert, union organizer, "Something New" (1973)

Labor organizing among women clerical workers occurred as far back as the 1900s; despite a lack of interest in organizing women clerical workers within established unions, a small number of women organized themselves, first through mutual benefit societies and later through unionism with the help of the Women's Trade Union League in the 1910s.[9] The 1920s saw a decline in organizing until the 1930s, when the largest clerical union, the United Office and Professional Workers of America (UOPWA), affiliated with the Congress of Industrial Organizations (CIO), was established. When it refused to release the names of its communist members, the UOPWA was expelled by the CIO in 1949.[10] As a result, the UOPWA folded. Through the 1950s and 1960s both office unionism and feminism became distant to women office workers. It was not until the resurgence of feminism, in the form of the women's liberation movement of the 1970s, that women office workers began organizing again.

Like the broader feminist movement, the women office workers' movement that emerged from it was not a single coherent entity. It was made up of scattered cells that had independently sprung up in cities sprinkled around the nation. On International Women's Day in 1971, at a National Organization of Women (NOW) conference in San Francisco, a handful of working class women formed their own feminist organization, Union WAGE. In Chicago, Women Employed was established. In Cleveland, Working Women. In New York, Women Office Workers (WOW). In Boston in 1972, two secretaries at Harvard's School of Education, Ellen Cassedy and Karen Nussbaum, formed 9to5, which held its first meetings in a room at the Cambridge YWCA.[11] Similar grassroots organizations were created in other cities. *Ms.* magazine reported that women's caucuses were even appearing in companies like Polaroid, Blue Cross, General Electric, and AT&T.[12] Critiques of the technologies and scientific management practices composing the late-capitalist office were central to this fledgling grassroots movement.

The office workers' movement was a new kind of labor activism. First, its founders envisioned their efforts as a practical extension of the larger women's movement into the lives and concerns of working-class women, allowing them to organize around gender instead of class. Second, the movement was formed of organizations independent of the male-dominated labor unions. The founders considered their efforts an innovation within the labor movement, providing women, many of whom had misgivings about unionism, with an alternative vehicle for responding to inequalities in the workplace. For example, 9to5 saw its role within the labor movement as "working on issues of discrimination and fair employment in general, developing activists in the cause of working women, and serving as a lightning rod for the expression of problems and concerns."[13] Feminism provided a means to reach and organize women across the nation around broad issues, even when their workplaces were not amenable to unionization. Though the founders of the office workers' movement were feminists and the membership almost entirely female, not all the women 9to5 tried to organize would have called themselves "feminists." Yet these women had been affected by the ideas of the women's movement, believing that they were due equal pay and respect. In response to many office workers' ambivalent relationship to feminism, organizers within the women office workers' movement exclusively focused on issues pertaining to working women, declining to take positions on such issues as abortion and sexuality.[14] Moreover, the women office workers' movement only organized those women who worked with information technologies, entirely neglecting other groups of women who worked in office buildings, such as cleaners, custodial workers, cafeteria workers, mailroom sorters, and so on. These workers, often new immigrants or women of color, remained invisible to and excluded from the movement, despite the occupational health hazards they faced in the same building.

The women office workers' movement was not by any means anti-union. However, it did feel a need to develop techniques outside of the traditional union drive that would speak to women who, though perhaps not feminists themselves, were living in the context of feminism. To this end, the women office workers' movement both drew on the agency feminism had granted women and imported tactics from feminism for its own grassroots organizing. In particular, the technique of "conscious-ness raising" became a crucial tool of the movement, used to convince women office workers that they had "rights" and deserved "respect" in the workplace, thereby paving the way for possible unionization.

Consciousness Raising

Consciousness raising, which had begun among radical feminists in New York in the late 1960s, spread rapidly across America.[15] By the end of 1970, every major city in the country had consciousness-raising groups—New York City alone had hundreds.[16] Even liberal feminist organizations like NOW were founding consciousness-raising groups. Consciousness raising was a discursive instrument: small groups of women got together, "rapped," shared their "experiences," found com-monalties, and began to analyze them in a discussion. It was a powerful technique for translating seemingly idiosyncratic personal events and emotions into a gender-based "experience."

Consciousness raising can be thought of as a technique for unsaying what has already been said ("the office works efficiently and safely") and saying what was unsaid ("the office is an exploitative and harmful tech-nology for extracting labor"). It was a technique for undoing the self-evidence of what might otherwise appear to be a fixed or natural social structure. It was also a technique that operated by collecting variation and turning it into commonality—it took accounts of different women's lives and abstracted a common womanness or class membership. This ability to produce an analysis based on a commonality underneath varia-tion assumed its own universalized subject—Woman with a capital W. Thus, consciousness raising functioned first by valorizing variation and then by covering it over. The use of consciousness raising by the women office workers' movement, moreover, depended precisely on this prob-lematic ability to transform difference into commonality.

Women Office Workers (WOW) of New York was founded through consciousness-raising techniques in the summer of 1973:

> Several office workers got together to rap about what could be done to improve the life of clerical workers. Some of us were active in the wom-en's organizations and some in unions. . . . we also believe[d] that office

workers are not immune to the consciousness raising that has been changing the lives of professional and middle-class women. What was missing was a vehicle for bringing together women office workers who often felt alienated from what went on at typical women's movement meetings.[17]

wow advertised its consciousness-raising sessions in its newsletter: "If you want to find out more about wow, we can come to your home to talk to you and your co-workers. It's sort of a Tupperware party idea, except we're not selling pans—we're exchanging experiences and ideas."[18] Similarly, Karen Nussbaum advised women in the *Working Woman's Guide to Office Survival*: "Suppose the office workers at your company have no organized group and you would like to start one . . . where do you begin? If your office chair is uncomfortable and the woman at the next desk has complained that her chair is also uncomfortable, then chances are you have already begun. Organizing begins when two or more people exchange common needs or grievances."[19]

The successful Hollywood movie *9 to 5* (1980) even brought consciousness raising to the masses. During a pivotal scene its stars, Jane Fonda, Lily Tomlin, and Dolly Parton, play disgruntled office workers who, encouraged by smoking marijuana one evening, begin to exchange experiences in a consciousness-raising session, realize their common oppression, and plot comic revenge.[20]

Through consciousness raising "experience" played a critical role in feminist analysis and was more generally an important referent in many political movements of the 1960s and the 1970s; it was mobilized as a counterknowledge that could set into question and even replace other types of expertise.[21] "Experience" was considered by radical feminists to be an alternate and more accurate source of knowledge about the status of women than already existent, male-produced knowledge, including scientific knowledge. Kathie Sarachild, the member of New York Radical Women who coined the term *consciousness raising*, argued that by basing their methods in experience, members of her group "were in effect repeating the seventeenth-century challenge of science to scholasticism: 'study nature, not books,' and put all theories to the test of living practice and action."[22] Consciousness raising was thus conceived as a successor science with better truth-telling capacities.

When consciousness raising was practiced in the women's health movement, "experience" became a type of personal knowledge originating in the body itself, and women were encouraged to trust their own corporeal sensations over medical authority. Thus, feminists tended to claim an epistemic privilege for experiential and embodied knowledge. It was possible, therefore, for some feminists to argue that the nature of oppression could only be accurately comprehended by the oppressed (and thus that no one else could refute their assertions). As members of a cultural elite, so the argument went, male scientists, sociologists, and managers were alienated from this knowledge gained through life under oppression. Thus, not only did appeals to experience bring political struggles down to the level of the body, they also asserted that oppression and suffering themselves provided special access to a type of knowledge that other expertise overlooked.

"Experience" is a category of knowledge that is just as historical as other forms of knowledge. The claim being made here is not as straightforward as asserting that our experiences of the world are shaped by culture and history. Instead, I am drawing attention to a stronger point: It is only through particular methods rooted historically in time and space that "experience" becomes a kind of evidence imbued with certain truth-telling qualities. Put more specifically, with the method of consciousness raising, "experience" of the intimate and minute details of one's personal life, and even one's body, became a kind of evidence of more general gendered phenomena. The persuasive force of the evidence of "experience" came from its being marked as (rather than self-evidently being) more proximate or "authentic" than expert knowledge. In short, in consciousness raising "experience" was not just collected, it was generated as a kind of evidence.

Oppression in the Details

With the aid of consciousness raising, practitioners transformed individual women's "experiences" into an analysis of the accumulation of small, trivial, day-to-day behaviors that made patriarchy possible and which, in turn, patriarchy constituted as invisible. It was this apprehension of how power operated through the details that connected women's bodies to the material conditions of office work. Feminist labor activists argued that oppression in the office was not necessarily obvious—women worked in air-conditioned rooms with potted plants and modern technological conveniences; rather, oppression took place in the seemingly trivial details of day-to-day interactions.[23] While designers promoted the plush carpets and modern furniture of the information economy as "humanity in an age of machines,"[24] feminist workers identified these same attributes as microtactics: "An older man sitting behind a huge oak desk in a large room with pictures on the wall of him shaking hands with President Nixon or John F. Kennedy, and his secretary at his side, uses all of that to intimidate. . . . One of these guys *starts off* by referring to you as girls, by intentionally forgetting your name and making sure that you know his. People now understand these things as *tactics* and they are willing to develop their own tactics to counterbalance his."[25] The subtle signals and daily minuscule humiliations—the way yellow and orange walls were meant to make workers feel "up," the way partitions isolated workers from each other, the way plastic modular furniture systems were advertised as a means to "solve your people problems,"[26] the way women had to fetch coffee—all these tiny details as construed by consciousness raising comprised the dispersed operation of office oppression.[27]

In 1977 the dispersed pockets of women activists began joining together to become a national group based in Cleveland, at first called Working Women, and then renamed 9to5 in 1983. By the early 1980s the movement had locals in Los Angeles, Baltimore, Boston, Minneapolis, Atlanta, Philadelphia, Washington, Pittsburgh, Cincinnati, Cleveland, Dayton, Providence, Seattle, San Francisco, and New York, with a total of over ten thousand members. As the movement grew and became more institutionalized, the grassroots technique of consciousness raising fell away, but the materialization of office oppression as occurring in the details remained. Following feminism's lead, the office workers' movement began to ask how the dispersed quality of office oppression might inscribe itself directly on the body, producing material effects that could be called occupational illness.

The Toxic Office

From its inception, the women office workers' movement was critical of the effects of automation and new digital technologies.[28] While desktop computers were not part of the office landscape until the 1980s, many back-office workers already were toiling on manual tasks affiliated with the computerization of office work. In the 1970s, an office worker might, for example, enter data on a VDT. An office worker also might work with a photocopier, which by the 1970s was standard office equipment. Not all new technologies were machines: carbonless paper and correction fluid had become common parts of office work, as had furniture made out of plastic, synthetic textiles, and chipboard. The budding environmental movement of the 1970s supported suspicion about hidden toxic chemicals, especially following incidents like that at Love Canal, where working-class women showed that supposedly ordinary neighborhoods were toxic, providing a new critical way of looking at everyday technologies and environments. Though the feminist office workers' movement made no explicit political alignment with the environmental movement, it is not surprising that office workers began to examine with suspicion the new technologies that made up the ordinary environment of the office: "No one knows much about the new machines being introduced as large offices automate or the chemical products that have replaced the old rubber eraser and typewriter brush. They smell bad, but just how much harm will they do over a period of years?"[29] Much suspicion was concentrated on the VDT: not only was it tied to concerns about automation and routinization, but workers who spent hours staring at a small green-on-black screen also ended up with eyestrain, headaches, and cramped necks. In cartoons from the early years of the office workers' movement, VDTS were sometimes portrayed as colonizing workers bodies, turning flesh into machine by virtue of the repetitive manual labor they required (see Fig. 12). Sitting inches away from a terminal, some women also wondered if low-level radiation emissions might cause miscarriages or otherwise damage their reproductive abilities.[30]

Jeanne Stellman was one of the few occupational health researchers in this period to be interested in the idea that the office could be hazardous to workers' health.[31] At conferences and meetings held by the feminist office workers' movement, Stellman was often the lone speaker on occupational health. In 1978 Stellman founded the Women's Occupational Health Resource Center in Brooklyn, New York, which served as a clearinghouse for information on women's occupational health issues and for a time became the center of feminist occupational-health efforts. Between 1981 and 1983 the resource center held training sessions for over four thousand workers, published a newsletter, and produced fact sheets (many based on Stellman's book) some of which covered the dangers of photocopiers, indoor air, VDT work, and other occupational hazards. Fact sheets typically listed a hazard and suggested a means of prevention. For example, the general fact sheet on "clerical work" published in 1980 listed excessive sitting, fatigue, stress, noise, poor office design, ozone, and organic solvents as the most prevalent office hazards. Above the list was the following caveat: "The exact nature and extent of office hazards are not known. They vary from office to office."[32] Since no rigorous scientific or epidemiological studies had yet connected a hazard with a specific occupational illness, Stellman's fact sheets were primarily speculative suggestions based on chemical ingredients also found in industrial settings. She justified her extrapolation from industrial exposures to the office setting by observing that, "today all workers have—in one way or another—become chemical workers and everybody is exposed to chemicals in the workplace."[33]

Encouraged by the suggestive statements in Stellman's work, 9to5 more carefully considered office technologies and quickly found that workers were surrounded by products that contained potentially toxic chemicals. Though these chemicals were usually present in minute quantities, no one had investigated their cumulative effect. Framing the effects of the office in terms of occupational health created a vehicle for connecting "the body"—the pivotal site of feminist politics—to office work. By 1980 occupational health became a core issue for 9to5, and Project Health and Safety was founded.

Project Health and Safety began by researching some of the chemicals that went into office technologies and building materials. It found reports that photocopier toner was linked to cancer.[34] It cited the testimony of one woman who had successfully filed a workers' compensation claim for exposure to photocopier exhaust.[35] It unearthed a handful of instances where office workers had suffered from formaldehyde poisoning and noted that the federal government was considering banning urea formaldehyde foam insulation.[36] Correction fluid also fell under the project's suspicion after newspapers reported that a Texas teenager died by using it as an inhalant (see Fig. 13).

Despite this research, Project Health and Safety did not collect enough evidence to launch a campaign around any specific technology, chemical, or illness associated with office work. Rather, what it had assembled was a sense that possible toxic exposures lurked everywhere, even in the most

Figure 12. Cartoons from the women office workers' movement of the 1970s often commented on the bodily and psychic effects of routinized data-processing labor done on early computing terminals. Here, the worker's body is colonized by the machinery of the VDT. From Tepperman, *Sixty Words a Minute*.

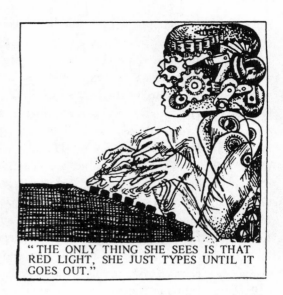

"THE ONLY THING SHE SEES IS THAT RED LIGHT, SHE JUST TYPES UNTIL IT GOES OUT."

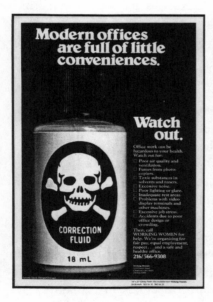

Figure 13. This poster from Project Health and Safety aptly expressed the view that dangers lurked in the tiniest details of office work. It also captures the way informal surveys—here a list of prompts to "watch out for"—were used for consciousness raising. Poster, Working Women, 1981.

seemingly banal of office supplies and technologies. The fact that these potential hazards were barely discernable made them, not more benign, but, as Ellen Cassedy explained, "all the more severe because they are often invisible and unrecognized." Nussbaum, quoted at length here, aptly captured this perception that insidious hazards lurked in the most unsuspecting places in the following excerpt from a speech:

> Let me give you a guided tour of the hazards in just sending out one letter:
>   Alice prepares to type a letter for Mr. Big. The carbonless typing paper she uses is made with abietic acid to fill the pores, and PCB's—polychlorinated by-phenyls. Abietic acid has been found to cause dermatitis and PCB's are extremely toxic, causing irritation to eyes, skin, nose and throat, can cause severe liver damage, and are suspected carcinogens. The typing ribbon she uses also contains PCB's.
>   To correct an error she uses a correction fluid containing trichloroethylene—TCE. In high doses, TCE can have a depressing effect on the central nervous system and can cause liver damage and lung dysfunction. . . . Alice goes to make a copy of the letter on the photocopy machine, which may emit ozone, a deadly substance. In poorly ventilated areas it's not hard to raise ozone to at least twice the federal standard. That black powder in the machine—the toner—may have nitropyrene or TNF, trinitroflourenone—suspected mutagens. . . . While in the copying room, Alice breathes methanol from the duplicating machine, which can cause liver damage. She ends her hazardous journey by filing Mr. Big's copy of the letter in a plastic file containing polyvinyl chloride, which can cause skin lesions and dermatitis.[37]

In other words, like office oppression, toxicity was in the details. To complicate matters further, these details varied from office to office and their health effects from person to person.

The women at Project Health and Safety understood that their conception of office occupational health was problematic and hard to believe (and that getting through to some managers might require extraordinary means, as caricatured in Fig. 14). Medical diagnosis, workers' compensation standards, and juridical precedent demanded more specific and acute causal explanations. As Stellman explained, "There is no disease currently known as officeitis, nor is there likely to be one. One can explain this by considering that each of the occupational health hazards . . . usually produce[s] a slow, subtle, insidious effect over time for which cause and effect may not be discernible. . . . In essence, the development

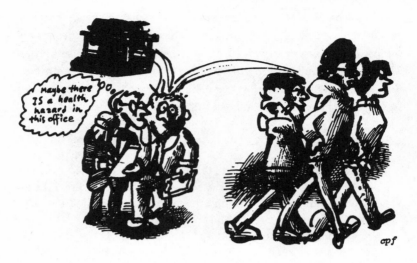

Figure 14. Management's disbelief in office hazards was a frequent theme in cartoons from the women office workers' movement in the 1970s. In this cartoon from the San Francisco–area group Union WAGE, workers literally hit management over the head with the reality of health hazards. From *Union Wage Newsletter*, April/May 1975.

of similar symptoms from many different low-level causes makes all chronic disease particularly difficult to understand."[38]

The obstacles to clinical recognition of nonspecific occupational health problems were numerous. Most physicians were trained to search for discrete disease entities, and there was no "officeitis." Further, since they diagnosed workers one at a time, doctors had difficulty perceiving building-wide patterns that consciousness raising might have revealed. Finally, the vague and often mild symptoms women workers presented could be explained by other diagnoses that medicine had developed long ago—"dysmenorrhea," "hysteria," or "psychosomatism" —and then treated with tranquilizing pharmaceuticals. In contrast to feminists, most doctors did not consider women's self-described experiences to be the most accurate registers of their health.

Additionally, occupational health investigators at the National Institute of Occupational Safety and Health (NIOSH) were not particularly concerned with office occupational health issues; the hazards of office work paled next to those industrial workers endured. When NIOSH investigators did examine office conditions, they usually came away empty-handed—their instruments, designed to register high levels of toxic chemicals in industrial settings, found no significant exposures to record in the office. Not only was a physical phenomenon imperceptible through their techniques, but the nonspecific phenomena officer workers complained of failed to fit the toxicological model of specific and acute chemical exposure and thus seemed outside the realm of possibility. Investigators at NIOSH found themselves turning to psychosomatic explanations, such as mass hysteria and mass psychogenic illness (MPI), to make sense of the variety and nonspecificity of women office workers' complaints.[39] Perhaps, some investigators suggested, such symptoms were a gendered psychological response to life stresses.

Surveys and "Experience"

Project Health and Safety needed a tool suited to its new institutionalized activism, one that could do some of the work consciousness raising had done when the movement had been more grassroots. Its activists needed a tool that could gather into a single event an unwieldy constellation of health effects, a tool that was affordable and easy to use without experts, a tool, unlike consciousness raising itself, that could transport their controversial vision of occupational health beyond themselves to persuade others. Here they turned to the survey.

In the 1980s, 9to5 increasingly left one-on-one organizing to union drives and focused on articulating—to workers, government, and the media—the broad issues that women office workers shared. Likewise, Project Health and Safety became concerned with occupational health, not to organize individual workplaces but to educate workers and authorities about the broader issue. The survey, imported from the social sciences, joined the grassroots feminist methods that had given birth to the movement. The power of the survey was that it performed several functions. For 9to5, it was important that the survey work as an extension of consciousness raising by other means. It had to compel workers to ask probing questions about their own bodies and surroundings. It had to continue the work of assembling dispersed experiences into a pattern of endemic oppression.[40] Of equal importance was the survey's ability to transport this apprehension to the media, to governments, and to expert audiences. While the survey performed these functions well, it also came into conflict with the appeal of consciousness raising to "experience" as a counterknowledge that could challenge expert knowledge and reductive science. The survey came with a price—it changed "experience" into quantitative evidence.

This change in the place of "experience" partially resulted from the institutional character of 9to5, which now had an executive board composed of members who chaired committees, a staff director who in turn hired other staff, and an executive director, Karen Nussbaum. No longer was the movement formed of office workers getting together at informal gatherings likened to "Tupperware parties." Instead, it was run by professional activists, mostly white and college-educated, who found themselves lobbying politicians, giving lecture tours, and testifying at congressional hearings.[41] The members of Project Health and Safety were no longer directly compelled by their own first-hand experiences of working in the office. For the career activist, the survey gathered the "experience" of office work at a distance; the social science survey already had a long tradition of such use by educated, feminist social workers. In the opening decades of the twentieth century, progressive social activists like those at Hull House and the influential industrial hygienist Alice Hamilton had innovatively used the social science survey in their work, participating in a British-U.S. Progressive Era social survey movement.[42] Surveys, administered by social workers, doctors, or union organizers, gathered information about the distribution of problems and capacities among the people one meant to help. The survey was a technology middle-class activists used to assess the conditions of others, especially the working class.

The survey, however, was not simply a vehicle for gathering information, it was a tool that 9to5 used to construct a nonspecific health event by gathering that information. In other words, Project Health and Safety already speculated about the nonspecificity of office occupational health and the survey was a means to congeal this apprehension for others. The surveys Project Health and Safety used came in a variety of forms: some were large and others small, some were used to gather statistical data and others were sent out for their consciousness-raising effects alone, some were administered by Project Health and Safety and others were designed for workers to administer to each other in their own office buildings. The first large survey conducted by Project Health and Safety was funded by an OSHA grant in 1981. It was distributed to eight thousand workers in the Boston and Cleveland areas, thirteen hundred of whom responded. The survey asked a hodgepodge of questions, covering such topics as stress levels, air quality, office environment, and office machines.[43] Its intent was not to uncover a particular disease or common problem underneath the variety of symptoms. Rather the survey was used to constitute the "nature" of office occupational illness—its diverse symptoms and varying conditions—by aggregating complaints into a single narrative and location. Thus surveys became not simply a way of gathering a diversity of information but a script through which diversity was arranged to illustrate a certain way of thinking about occupational health. On the heels of Project Health and Safety's work followed the publication of several popular books on office hazards, each appended by a comprehensive survey which workers could use to assess their own work conditions.[44] A survey distributed in a particular office building was sometimes used explicitly to organize workers around the conditions found there, sparking what came to be called "sick building" episodes.

While a survey could be used to make a sick building episode perceptible and then organize workers around it, the survey's power to transport "experience" outside the movement came from its ability to objectify and quantify.[45] With the survey, workers no longer actually had to talk to each other about their "experiences," instead they could anonymously check off predetermined categories on a sheet of paper. These anonymous responses were then tabulated to create a statistical profile. The survey need not uphold strict standards of scientific rigor to be effective; the statistical format of the survey was usually sufficient to signal a scientistic "objective" measure. By objectifying and quantifying, surveys translated the nonspecific nature of office pathology into a scientistic format and bureaucratic language socially invested with the power to measure and give shape to the material. With the survey, "experience" was turned from a naturalized "counterknowledge" into evidence to be analyzed with quantitative methods. In the process, the voices of workers were transformed, as was their claim to comprehend oppression more fully, to be replaced by a genre more palatable to the bureaucrat and better able to mobilize government resources. Thanks to surveys, a host of impressive numbers were now at 9to5's disposal. A congressman on the U.S. House Committee on Energy and Commerce could be told that "70% of the office workers surveyed complained of severe indoor pollution, poor circulation, and irritating fumes."[46] Or a press release might announce that "4 out of 5 workers describe their jobs as somewhat or very stressful."[47] Project Health and Safety widely publicized the results of its surveys on the radio, in newspapers, at congressional hearings, and medical conferences. At the level of the building, a survey could be used to provoke a NIOSH Health Hazard Investigation.

Thus the survey became a powerful technology for making nonspecific problems perceptible to workers, management, and government experts. Unlike the air samplers, X-rays, and other instruments used by conventional occupational health investigations, surveys were able to capture a phenomenon that was nonspecific and only discernable in a cluster, not in an individual. This assemblage of gendered subjects, "experience," surveys, nonspecificity, and commonality out of variation created its own domain of imperception. It was incapable of detecting the kinds of causal proof workers' compensation boards demanded. Surveys could only materialize the contours and expression of an occupational health phenomenon, not the causes behind it. Thus the survey left unresolved the lingering question of whether office occupational health had psychological or material origins.

Stressed Out

In 1982, Project Health and Safety administered a large "Stress Test," distributing over forty thousand surveys largely through women's magazines.[48] The Stress Test, like 9to5's first survey, asked many questions, listing thirty-four possible sources of stress (including rate of promotion, deadlines, keystroke quotas, isolation, and sexual remarks) and signs of stress (high blood pressure, smoking, heart disease, miscarriages, and nervous agitation). Again, the survey was not intended to whittle stress down to a few well-delimited expressions. Instead it spread the effects and sources of stress as widely as possible, thereby constituting the capillary nature of office occupational health. These large surveys were then supplemented by small, self-administered surveys at meetings, in Project Health and Safety's newsletter, and in women's magazines in order to elicit a consciousness-raising effect.

Project Health and Safety's portrait of "toxicity in the details" was becoming complicated by the group's desire to expand the scope of workplace assaults from chemical exposures to nonphysical social assaults. The term "stress" encapsulated this view that dispersed and chronic office exploitation manifested itself in bodily symptoms. "Stress," however, was a polyvalent term whose meaning the movement could not control. Project Health and Safety had to carefully negotiate the quagmire surrounding articulations of stress, for "hysteria" and "psychosomaticism" were psychological explanations closely tied to it. "Stress" was always in danger of being swallowed by "hysteria," a term used to explain away often vague physical symptoms as simply the result of a gender-based psychological disposition, perhaps even rooted in menstruation, rather than a response to adverse work conditions.[49]

Instead of granting stress a psychological foundation, feminist office activists wanted to couple stress tightly with the late-capitalist information age. "If loss of limb and back pain are the characteristic hazards of the industrial age," explained Karen Nussbaum, "then job stress is the characteristic hazard of the computer age. It's an insidious hazard, because it's hard to identify and as Americans we frown on what we consider to be a personality weakness. But stress is not in your head, it's in the office. And it could be a blight on society."[50] Stress still proved a slippery subject to define. Union WAGE described stress in vague terms as something that "cannot be measured the way the noise level or temperature can be and is connected to workers having some control over their working conditions."[51] How could one measure stress? How could one avoid its dismissal as an individual's psychological inability to cope with the pressures of the workplace?

The link between stress and office work was confirmed for activists in a series of epidemiological studies that lent their claims scientific credence. In 1975 NIOSH reported that office workers had the second highest incidence of stress-induced diseases of any occupational group, and in 1980 it stated that VDT workers had the highest stress levels ever recorded.[52] The Framingham Heart Study provided further evidence, calculating that women office workers developed heart disease at a rate two times that of other women workers.[53] Project Health and Safety activists were willing to point to these studies to lend credence to their claims, but they were not willing to accept the often accompanying analysis that stress was rooted in a gendered psychology. They mobilized a two-pronged strategy for explaining stress in nonpsychological terms: stress was a *biological* reaction to *social* conditions.

By pointing to social causes, office activists were using stress to argue for the necessity of restructuring office work. The members of the short-lived Nasty Secretaries Liberation Front (who later published *Processed World*) costumed themselves as computer terminals while handing out leaflets on stress to office workers in San Francisco. The pamphlet insisted that "stress is a social disease and it has a social cure . . . Stress is not a result of individual failings. It is the result of an irrational and inhumane society. The solution to stress will not be found in any special seminar or in any special meditation or exercise techniques. . . . it will take a deliberate restructuring of the social order to reduce it in any real sense."[54]

What elements of the "social order" should be restructured? The litany of social and work factors contributing to stress in the office were endless and diffuse. Every facet of workplace conditions was involved: from environmental quality issues (temperature and overcrowding) to labor relations (lack of respect and no promotions) to job design (constant sitting and repetitive work). Stress was the expression of the dispersed quality of office oppression, and thus its presence revealed failures of the social order, not the worker.

The proof of "stress," for feminist office activists, was in workers' bodies: shaky hands, headaches, nervous stomach, high blood pressure, ulcers, and menstrual-cycle irregularities, any of which led many women to turn to pharmaceuticals to get through the day. This corporeal evidence was accounted for by pointing to an underlying nonpathological biological mechanism that translated adverse social conditions into biological expressions; borrowing from the modern stress theory of Hans Selye the feminist office movement called on a biologically based "General Adaptation" response.[55] Jeanne Stellman, for example, explained stress in the following fashion: "We can think of the stress response as a mechanism for adapting to the environment. In fact, some scientists call the stress response the general adaptation syndrome, . . . the body responds to different inputs in an identical manner."[56] In other words, the causes of stress were nonspecific, but their effects on the body accumulated in a general way and could be seen in the bodily symptoms of stress. In its newsletter, 9to5 described stress similarly: stress is "the body's way of protecting itself from physical, mental, or emotional strain. Heart and breathing rates increase, muscles tighten, and stomach acid and adrenaline are released. After a brief stressful incident, the body quickly returns

Figure 15.
The office workers' movement and other critical commentators, such as Chris Carlson of the San Francisco zine *Processed World*, the artist who created this illustration (1981), portrayed stress as a normal biological reaction to an oppressive workplace. Courtesy of *Processed World*, www.processed-world.com.

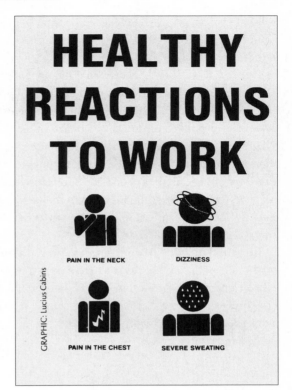

GRAPHIC: Lucius Cabins

to a balanced state. But constant stressful demands keep the body off balance, creating symptoms such as headaches, nervousness and fatigue. Prolonged stress can cause serious illnesses like high blood pressure and coronary heart disease."[57] Through such descriptions, feminist labor activists attempted to show that stress was a normal biological reaction, rather than a pathological, psychological one: stress was not the result of an abnormal individual's psyche but a normal response to unhealthful conditions (see Fig. 15).

The meanings circulating under "stress," however, were impossible to fix under this two-pronged strategy. In the late 1970s and in the 1980s, the term was used widely to describe the anxiety of living in the late twentieth century.[58] Popularly, and in contradistinction to the NIOSH studies, stress was most often associated with elite jobs: executives, careerists, and professionals. A stress industry blossomed catering to the stressed-out, high-income market, providing hordes of advice, self-help books, exercise, hobbies, diets, and biofeedback therapies. The self-help industry around stress focused on changing the individual, rather than social conditions.

Even feminist labor activists had difficulty entirely avoiding individualistic accounts of stress. Their own advice had a tendency to fade into platitudes indistinguishable from popular rhetoric. While 9to5's *The Working Woman's Guide to Office Survival* noted that the only real solution to stress was to eliminate its sources through workplace organizing, the majority of its advice and column inches were dedicated to visualizing, stretching, dieting, hobbies, and expressing yourself.[59] Office-related stress was even included in a chapter of *Jane Fonda's Workout Book*—a succinct expression of feminism as self-discipline rather than social change.[60]

Stress remained a risky diagnosis. Yet the claim that the dispersed quality of office oppression was materially revealed in the biology of office workers was a radical twist.[61] Bodies did not react only to low-level chemical exposures but also to unjust social factors. Through the survey, 9to5 captured these bodily reactions while leaving their causes dispersed and open.

Toward Sick Building Syndrome

There is still no single "disease" associated with office work. Instead of finding a shared affliction such as black lung or silicosis, the women office workers' movement materialized a nonspecific phenomenon that clashed with juridical, medical, and compensatory institutional demands for proof of linear causality. The women office workers' movement was only able to capture the symptomatic expression of workplace conditions by simultaneously leaving the question of their causal root uncertain. Despite this dilemma, the women office workers' movement was effective in rendering perceptible a new kind of occupational health event that workers could, and would, organize around later—sick building syndrome.

Sick building syndrome was not a "disease" at all but was defined by occupational health experts as a phenomenon that manifested as a multitude of symptoms, mostly minor, associated with a particular office building and for which no single cause could be found. The symptoms associated with sbs not only varied from episode to episode, they changed from worker to worker within a single episode. Moreover, the proof of sick building syndrome was not in a blood test, air monitor, petri dish, or other form of "objective" scientific measure; it lay in the density of worker complaints, first as expressed through worker protests and later as captured by experts' surveys. The numerous grassroots protests around individual problem buildings kept the issue of office occupational health in the limelight.

The phenomenon of sick building syndrome, however, has developed in contexts quite different from those generated by the women office workers' movement. With the dramatic rise of unionism in the public sector and a corresponding greater willingness to organize women by established organizations like the AFL-CIO, sick building syndrome has become untangled from the extra-union women office workers' movement and its feminist character. Karen Nussbaum became exemplary of the changed status of women office workers in unions—first, as head of the Women's Bureau in the U.S. Department of Labor in 1993, and then as director of the Working Women's Department at the AFL-CIO. She became the highest-ranking female official in the U.S. labor movement.[62] Though the rank and file of clerical unions might be female, sbs was rarely figured as a women's issue even though the role of gender in sbs was hotly debated among occupational health professionals and in courtrooms. Why did episodes primarily affect women? Did this indicate a gendered psychological cause? Was sbs caused by cumulative chemical exposure or mass hysteria?[63]

The emergence of office occupational health problems cannot be understood simply as the result of newly pathological workplace conditions or as the discovery of a previously hidden problem by experts, or even by workers. The problem was materialized by methods, tools, and actions assembled by workers that together made possible a kind of occupational health event otherwise unmaterialized. The problem could be materialized by office workers in the way it was because ventilation engineers, office designers, and corporate managers had already physically made office buildings into a certain kind of place. Through the assemblage put together by office workers, office health problems became a phenomenon about which things could be said and done.

Yet this materialization, like all others, carried its own set of constraints, for the assemblage of tools and practices the women office workers' movement used only performed in certain ways. On the one hand, while these activists articulated nonspecific health events, they could not connect bodies and work conditions in the terms of causality and specificity that health institutions conventionally demanded. On the other hand, by connecting office work to bodies primarily as health events, rather than as acts of oppressive labor conditions, the feminist office workers' movement unwittingly set the stage for the depoliticization of office occupational health events through the diagnosis of sick building syndrome. The next chapter examines in detail the coming into being of sick building syndrome in the clash between industrial hygiene experts and practitioners of popular epidemiology.

[4] **Break down a late-twentieth-century** office building into its array of mass-produced materials. The extent and variety of products amassed into the ubiquitous, square office building are astounding. Sprays of rustproofing and fire retardant cling to steel-girder skeletons. Plastic-sheathed wires and sealant-coated ducts snake amid a rainbow of insulation fibers. Formaldehyde and adhesive preserve and hold fast plywood and fiberboard veneers. At the end of the millennium, building materials were more likely to come from a manufacturer's cauldron than from a tree or a stone.

Take ever present office carpet, for example, churned out in batches extending millions of square feet. Carpet plush, made out of nylon, polyester, or polypropylene, was not woven but seared onto a latex rubber, polyvinyl chloride, or hydrocarbon resin backing with styrene butadiene, and then sprayed with fungicide, stain retardant, and fireproofing. Yet another solvent-based adhesive glued the carpet to the plywood subfloor. Each of the these elements—plush, backing, glues—were at some point in their manufacture a liquid stew of molecules, the exact ingredients of which were tinkered with in industry labs: styrene, 1,2-dichloroethane, ethyl benzene, toluene, 1,1,1-trichloroethane, and xylenes, to name just a few. Once unrolled, the seemingly solid carpet "off-gassed" whiffs of its constituent chemicals into the air. Molecules and tiny particulates escaped from the carpet and joined the air at a density thick enough to acquire a vernacular name, "new carpet smell," for what scientists call 4-phenylcyclohexene. The revolution in mass-produced synthetic building materials that began in the postwar era brought dramatic change to the built environment of daily life—in the words of DuPont's advertising campaign, "Better things for better living . . . through chemistry."

Perfumed workers, vapors from building materials, and office equipment fumes persistently contributed molecular constituents into the indoor atmosphere. The collection of molecules making up "air" inevitably entered the mouth and nose, passing into the trachea and then the lungs. Along with oxygen and carbon dioxide, other molecules—aerosols, volatile organic compounds, and other lipid soluble molecules—diffused across the wall of the alveoli into the blood. The molecules that made up new carpet smell merged into bodies. Smell is not like touch. It is not a meeting of two objects at the surface but a penetration into the body of ingredients once belonging to another object. The protagonists of this chapter—molecules and chemicals—depended on toxicologists and industrial hygienists, as well as workers, to make perceptible their journeys from environment to bodies.

In the 1980s and 1990s, thousands of workers in hundreds of American office buildings worried that they were exposed to harmful chemicals. With grievances and protests that often captivated local media, throngs of office workers instigated National Institute of Occupational Safety and Health (NIOSH) investigations. In its first seven years, from 1971–78, NIOSH only received six health hazard evaluations requests for nonindustrial buildings. From 1978 to 1980, the number grew to 115. And in the single year of 1988, there were eighty-six, or 22 percent of yearly health hazard evaluation requests.[1] During the 1980s, "indoor pollution" became an object of activism, investigation, and possible regulation, subtly linked to a growing movement to regulate public tobacco use. In 1984, Congress added indoor-pollution research to a reluctant EPA's mandate through a line item addition to the agency's budget. From 1987 to 1992, the fight against indoor pollution, championed by the environmentally minded congressman Joseph Kennedy (D-R.I.), became the subject of congressional hearings on a proposed Indoor Air Quality Act. The Congress's report quoted the declaration by the director of the Consumer Federation of America that indoor pollution was "the nation's number one hidden health threat."[2] In 1988, Philip Morris, R. J. Reynolds Tobacco Company, Lorillard Corporation, Svenska Tobaks AB, and Brown Williamson Tobacco Corporation together founded the nonprofit Center for Indoor Air Research (CIAR), which quickly became the largest nongovernmental source of funding for indoor air pollution research, supporting both reputable scientists at major universities and industry-supportive research on the effects of secondhand smoke.[3] While most office buildings over the course of the 1980s had become

nonsmoking spaces, tobacco companies hoped that the plethora of products contributing to indoor pollution would help take the spotlight off
cigarettes. As attention to indoor air grew, requests for NIOSH investigations of office buildings reached a peak of 814 for the single year of 1993,
or 71 percent of the all requests made to NIOSH.[4]

Chemical exposures were, and are, notoriously difficult to prove. They
are composed of molecules invisible to the unaided eye (if not the nose)
and are usually only investigated well after the initial moment of their
presence. In debates over incidents of chemical exposure, the difficulties
of objectively proving that errant molecule A, released at moment B,
caused symptoms x, y, and z have habitually thrown the very reality of
exposures into question. The uncertainty that clung to chemical exposures mired office occupational health complaints in the 1980s. When
government industrial hygienists arrived to investigate troublesome office buildings, their air samplers rarely detected any significant chemical
presence that might explain the multiplicity of symptoms of which flocks
of workers complained, from sinus infections to rashes and headaches.

The term *sick building syndrome* was first used in 1984 by a Danish-
born Yale biophysicist in a Swedish publication and quickly proliferated
in the English-language medical literature and in media accounts of
problem office buildings on both sides of the Atlantic.[5] The name was
immediately controversial—how could a building properly be called
"sick"?[6] Moreover, the events SBS described were themselves strange
in form—imperceptible chemical exposures combined with multiple
symptoms. Could such events be proved real? Were offices, homes,
schools, and malls—spaces previously understood as shelters from
hazard—polluted?

NIOSH investigators and other indoor-pollution researchers fell into
two camps, one arguing that indoor pollution existed in chronic and nonspecific forms and that sick building syndrome was a legitimate phenomenon, the other holding that sick building syndrome was a misnomer for
what was better understood as a gendered psychological delusion.

This chapter contrasts two different, historically specific ways scientists and workers materialized chemical exposures as discernable events
that were nonetheless uncertain and almost impossible to prove. Over
the course of the twentieth century, two distinct traditions, two distinct
regimes of perceptibility—what I will identify as toxicology and popular
epidemiology—characterized the effects of buildings on bodies in con-

flicting ways. I argue that sick building syndrome came into being with its uncertain and nonspecific form at the convergence of these two different ways of apprehending chemical exposures. Toxicology and popular epidemiology depended on different assemblages for perceiving exposures, thereby invoking discrepant terms for their existence.

As with ventilation engineering, the assemblages that governed both toxicology and popular epidemiology were simultaneously productive and constraining. Each allowed the apprehension of some qualities, attributes, and connections, but not others. Each of the two assemblages I trace involved a disengagement from a broader field of possibilities for the sake of focusing on, isolating, and rendering intelligible a more narrowly delineated set of qualities. Both assemblages, moreover, were infused with relations of gender and privilege. Throughout the twentieth century, feminist activists, investigators, and even bureaucrats drew attention to occupational health issues, while white women workers have been singled out for rescue and protection.[7] Performances of gender informed the very technologies, practices, and subject positions that composed both industrial hygiene and popular epidemiology. At stake in struggles to render chemical exposures perceptible then was not only how to observe errant molecules, but also who legitimately observed and who experienced exposures.

Toxicology, Industrial Hygiene, and Specificity

Solvents. Polycyclic Aromatic Hydrocarbons. Dibromochloropropane. Vinyl chloride. Acrylamide. Toluene Diisocyanate. Carbon Disulfice. Pentachlorophenol. Ethylene Oxide.—Table of contents, in Zenz, *Occupational Medicine*

Open up an occupational medicine textbook from the late twentieth century and the table of contents will likely read like a list of chemicals.[8] Each chemical has a threshold level value at which it becomes toxic and a description of the effects caused in the human body once that threshold is passed. There are no portraits of the factory floor or labor conditions. There are no tales of family hardship. Instead, these descriptions are written in a specialized language originating in laboratories, where the techniques of toxicology rendered industrial chemicals measurable. Crack open toxicology to find out how it connected chemicals to bodies.

Beginning in the eighteenth century with the work of the French chemist Antoine-Laurent Lavoisier, scientists apprehended that air was ordinarily composed of oxygen and carbon dioxide.[9] American ventilation engineers in the early twentieth century had concluded that the chemical constituents of ordinary air were largely irrelevant to human comfort or health in office buildings. Industrial hygienists, in contrast, were interested in the dangerous chemicals found in factory atmospheres.[10] That is, they were interested in chemicals emanating from the industrial landscape that were unnatural to air.

Alice Hamilton, one of the most influential founders of American industrial hygiene, straddled the social worlds of the laboratory and Progressive Era reform movements.[11] Hamilton, a doctor with advanced training in bacteriology and pathology, joined Jane Addams's Hull House settlement in Chicago, in which middle-class professional women, often feminists, lived among, studied, and served the poor, especially immigrants.[12] Instead of drawing on the rhetoric and strategies of organized labor, white middle-class women reformers mobilized maternalism to call for the protection of women of primarily European descent. In arguing for protectionist legislation, they strategically asserted that women possessed sex-specific biological frailties requiring special treatment. Moreover, they argued that women's dual roles as workers and mothers meant that industrial chemicals were not simply potential poisons but also what Hamilton called "race poisons."[13] From the inception of American industrial hygiene, the gender and race of workers was an important consideration.

Maternalist protectionist strategies grew out of what historian Allison Hepler has called an early-twentieth-century "environmentalist worldview" in which, first, sickness was caused by environmental conditions and, second, workplace conditions could be carried into the home, not by chemicals clinging to clothes, but rather by impeding women's important reproductive work for the family, the society, and the race. Protectionism, advocates of the Equal Rights Amendment pointed out, could function as a feint to "protect" women from the higher-paying jobs of male unionized workers.[14]

Though Hamilton used some laboratory methods in her investigations, they were only one tool in her larger array of techniques. She relied primarily on walk-through factory inspections and surveys of employees and local clinicians.[15] Using a social science methodology prac-

ticed at Hull House, she investigated workplaces and meticulously interviewed workers in their homes, learning their symptoms, measuring
lead levels on their clothes and in their kitchens, and convincing them to
disclose how management might be obstructing her investigation. It
was the knowledge of workers, foremen, and neighborhood doctors
garnered from years working with an industrial process that Hamilton
drew on in her inspections and surveys. It might be said, then, that her
success was due more to her personal persuasiveness and ability to write
heart-rending portraits of factory life than to the objectivity of the science
she wielded.

While the expectation that the government should provide information about the safety of workplace chemicals arose in the Progressive
Era, it was not until the interwar years that the assemblage of technologies, people, and practices that gave shape to contemporary regulatory toxicology was first articulated.[16] With the "red scare" that immediately followed the First World War and the Russian Revolution, the
reformist and radical politics of the Progressive Era were severely re-
pressed. The ascendant conservative patriotism brought with it violent
suppression of strikes and the deportation of foreign-born radicals. In
this repressive context of the early 1920s, organized labor declined in
strength and so too did progressive and radical agitation around occupational health. It was also in this period that scientific industrial hygiene
gained its first institutional foothold with the establishment of university
laboratories. At prestigious schools such as Harvard, Yale, Johns
Hopkins, Columbia, and the University of Pennsylvania, industrial
hygiene labs offered an alternative to previous public health attempts to
police occupational disease through the use of surveys, inspections,
legislation, and physical examinations.[17] In contrast to Hamilton's
efforts to politicize her scientific work, industrial hygiene labs in the
interwar years offered their toxicological and physiological services to
companies as an objective, apolitical, and nonlegislative way to arbitrate
occupational disease disputes.[18]

Naively, perhaps, some university industrial hygienists expected that
the modern company would put the knowledge they gained from academic laboratory experiments into use without legislation—just because
it made for good business. They appealed to companies for funding,
selling themselves as neither prolabor nor proindustry but as an independent set of experts who could settle labor disputes over occupational

health equitably and without resort to politics. As the historian Christopher Sellers has shown, their professional power and political "independence" was founded on a move from the field to the lab and from humans to animals, a move that helped depoliticize their science.[19] Within the lab, success hinged on their technical ability to perceive what was invisible to the clinician or worker: the specific chain of effects that a chemical consistently caused in human physiology. That is, by passing the connection between chemicals and bodies through the laboratory, industrial hygiene promised to objectify the cause and result of industrial disease.

The industrial hygiene division at Harvard, founded in 1918, was one of the most important sites where the assemblage of industrial hygiene was set. In 1919, Hamilton joined the Harvard faculty, which included such notable scientists as Cecil Drinker, a physician turned physiologist who headed the new industrial hygiene research program, and Joseph Aub, known for his medical research into cancer, metabolism, and toxicology. The chemistry of disease was a central research concern at Harvard, influenced by the presence of the physiological chemist Lawrence J. Henderson, known for his pathbreaking studies of blood chemistry, and the influential physiologist Walter Cannon, who studied physiology in terms of chemical regulation and disequilibria. Henderson's career reveals the range of sympathies of Harvard's industrial hygiene: in addition to his work on chemistry, he was affiliated with the Harvard Business School, applying the insights he gained from physiology to management theory.[20]

How did toxicology connect work environments and workers' bodies? Industrial hygienists, with the help of their physiologist collaborators, engaged the human body, unsurprisingly, in terms of chemistry and chemical regulation. They developed techniques that could detect small amounts of a substance in the blood and used animal experiments to find the physiochemical mechanism that could account for the corresponding disease. The lead-poisoning research done at Harvard was the emblematic example: industrial hygienists could detect lead in the atmosphere, then in the blood and tissue, and finally could trace the specific set of physiochemical changes which lead regularly caused in the body.[21]

Core to this emergent field of toxicology were, first, the techniques of experimental physiology that could be practiced on animals; second, the instruments that measured physiological processes, rendering them quantitative, standardized, and thus comparative; and third, the exposure chamber, a technology that was imported from ventilation-engineering research. Ventilation research was as much a part of Harvard's industrial hygiene division as was toxicology. Cecil Drinker hired his brother Philip Drinker, an engineer involved with ventilation research at ASHVE and the inventor of the iron lung, to design an environmental chamber for use in chemical exposure experiments much like the chamber he constructed with Constantine Yaglou, also a faculty member in the division, for use in researching the comfort zone. Instead of using the sealed chamber to tinker with climatic variables, industrial hygienists introduced a specific chemical at a controlled concentration and measured its effects on their experimental subjects (see Fig. 16). At Harvard, the compounds studied included benzene, manganese, lead, radium, carbon monoxide, and sulfuric acid vapor. In 1938 the American Conference of Government Industrial Hygienists (ACGIH) formed and founded a committee to develop safety standards for industrial chemicals.[22] In 1946 it released its first list of what were then called "maximum allowable concentrations" (MACS), and refashioned in 1956 as "threshold limit values" (TLVS). This switch was not simply technical but also a move away from the Russian-used MAC in a rabidly anticommunist era.[23]

The first regime of perceptibility in this chapter's story was based on a material assemblage inscribed into the tools and practices of laboratory industrial hygiene and visually represented by the "dose-response curve" used to determine a TLV.[24] Here, when a body was placed within the "empty box" of the environmental chamber, it was not a white man's body but rather a mass-produced white rabbit, rat, or, more typically, a mouse, bred for its ability to react to chemicals in predictable ways. There was not just one box but several, each containing a group of around fifty animals, which were exposed to a different, fairly high dose of a chemical for about one-third of their lifetime—which calculates to just a matter of months for mice.[25] Toxicologists then detected those physiological changes that were, first, discernable with available diagnostic tests (of course, mice cannot speak for themselves), and, second, regular enough to occur numerous times in a small group of only fifty animals.

The number of animals in each box with health effects was then plotted in a graph against the concentration of the chemical exposure.

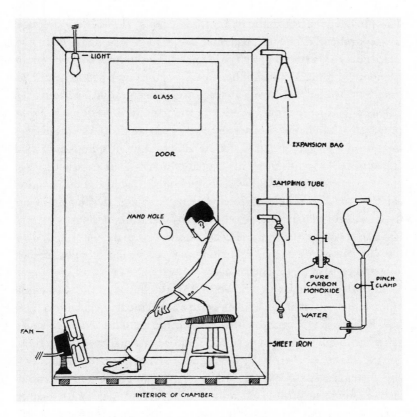

Figure 16. Line drawing from 1921 of an environmental chamber used to experimentally measure the effects of carbon monoxide on humans at the Yale Laboratory of Applied Physiology. The actual chamber was built of wood, covered in sheet iron, and hermetically sealed with plaster. Carbon monoxide was introduced through a tube. The effects on the test subject were measured by taking blood samples through the hand hole. From Yandell Henderson et al., "Physiological Effects," 85.

This provided the beginning of the dose-response curve. Every chemical had its own curve, but dose-response curves in general had a distinctive shape. Because experimenters used fairly high chemical concentrations in order to induce significant health effects, the curve had to be mathematically extrapolated downward for lower concentrations, allowing scientists to predict the concentration at which no health effects would be provoked. The chemical concentration at this point on the graph was then divided by one hundred, for an extra margin of safety, and called the "threshold limit value" for human workers daily exposed to that chemical at work five days a week, eight hours a day. These toxicological experiments were only concerned with materializing physiological reactions to chemicals that were both *regular*—that is, replicable—and *specific*—that is, a signature physiological reaction for that chemical. Bodies, likewise, were investigated as objects that reacted specifically, predictably, and consistently to chemicals.

In the decades following the Second World War, with the weakening of the industrial labor movement, occupational medicine fell from prestige. In the postwar period, toxicology became an independent specialty as its techniques and tools drifted from occupational disease to more general studies of chemicals, such as the testing of consumer products and pesticides. Toxicology labs were no longer run by famous physiologists or found at prestigious universities. Instead they had spread to bureaucracies like the Food and Drug Administration (FDA) and to private corporate research labs that became important fixtures of large American corporations in the 1950s and 1960s.[26] Companies no longer relied on the expertise of university industrial hygienists, instead testing their chemicals in-house, thereby ensuring greater control over the methods and results. The ACGIH began publishing its list of TLVs as voluntary standards in 1962 and has since published seven editions covering 642 substances (only a small fraction of the chemical ingredients used in manufacturing). Determining TLVs was expensive and time consuming. Most of the TLVs were based on suggestions made by chemical and manufacturing company representatives rather than by published or peer-reviewed research. Published TLVs were often based on not actual science but "consensus" among committee members, who included corporate toxicologists from DuPont, Dow, Bayer, and other chemical manufacturers, as well as equipment manufacturers.[27] An early chair of the ACGIH Threshold Limits Committee, Lawrence Fairhill, candidly revealed that the committee sought "values which, on the one hand, protect the individual workman, and on the other hand, impose no impossible burden on the manufacturer."[28] The point I want to make, however, is not that the research behind TLVs was suspect, sloppy, and corporate in origin (which it often was), but rather that even at its most rigorous, this method was highly constrained in what it could do and perceive.

This assemblage for materializing the effects of chemicals on bodies was highly successful, hence the successful association of lead to lead poisoning, silicon to silicosis, asbestos to asbestosis.[29] From the 1930s to the 1960s, specific diseases like silicosis were added incrementally to state workers' compensation schedules. Industrial hygiene, in turn, constructed instruments to use in the field—such as air samplers and blood tests—made to record acute levels of known chemicals in industrial settings and their signature physiological reaction. As workers' compensation boards and courts attempted to adjudicate disputes over chemical exposure, they, too, employed the standards of proof established by toxicology.[30] Slowly, by sporadic increments, state compensation programs covered any discrete occupational diseases for which the claimant could demonstrate (1) an exposure to a specific chemical, (2) the symptoms affiliated with exposure to that chemical, and (3) a blood test, X-ray, or other standardized diagnostic test which objectively demonstrated a physiological effect typical of that chemical. If they adhered to this form, chemical exposures were granted existence in juridical and medical realms. Workers seeking compensation were thus dependant on experts to materialize the effect of chemicals on their bodies.

This regime also produced a domain of imperceptibility. While toxicology was undoubtedly effective at rendering perceptible certain kinds of occupational disease, it simultaneously lent a narrow shape to what counted as a significant chemical exposure, creating a domain of imperceptibility where other reactions fell. Reactions to combinations of chemicals or to chronically low-level exposures, as well as rare or variable reactions all fell outside the practices of toxicology and industrial hygiene. The dominant assemblage in toxicology not only rendered perceptible the specific bodily effects of chemicals, it also set up criteria by which one could *exclude* a bodily condition from the category of occupational disease. While silicosis could be identified by X-rays, and lead poisoning by blood tests, other occupational illnesses failed to fit so easily into a diagnostic test.[31] When workers' symptoms failed to fit this mold, companies and compensation plans could persuasively claim that no occupational disease existed, or at least that financial compensation was not warranted. Lack of research on a particular disease, poor fit with approved diagnostic tests, or long-term effects that were not amenable to toxicological methods could all result in an occupational illness's remaining uncompensated and rendered imperceptible. In other words, the absence of specificity could be used to claim nonexistence. Low-level and mixed exposures became de facto uncertain phenomena.

Founded in 1971, NIOSH, charged with the task of researching and investigating occupational safety and health, and OSHA, the federal agency mandated to regulate the safety of workplaces, quickly and uncritically adopted TLVS as official standards for workplace air. When NIOSH investigated office buildings, their methods and tools, designed for industrial settings, could not help but reproduce this domain of imperceptibility.[32] Industrial air samplers almost always failed to perceive any sign of acute chemical exposure, and investigators could only find a multitude of seemingly unrelated symptoms. Published research into sick buildings bemoaned difficulties in detecting exposures: "extensive air sampling programs in a number of tight building syndrome investigations have yet to detect air contaminants at concentrations exceeding, or even approaching, any Threshold Limit Value."[33] Most researchers turned to poor ventilation as a catchall explanation. Even epidemiological research involving large samples and controls could find no specific chemical agent but only reduced ventilation rates in a sealed-window building.[34]

With no discernable chemical exposures and no discrete illness, NIOSH investigators had difficulty saying that anything physical was happening in office outbreaks. How then to account for complaints of chemical exposure?

Gendering Nonexistence

Psychologists at NIOSH and elsewhere began suggesting that perhaps these incidents were a form of mass psychogenic illness (MPI), also known as mass hysteria.[35] MPI was understood as a pathology of perception, a form of misperception in which workers wrongly attributed their symptoms to their physical workplace when the symptoms really had a psychological origin. The criteria for MPI, based on the *Diagnostic Statistic Manual* entry for psychosomatic disorder, was technically a diagnosis by exclusion: "the collective occurrence of physical symptoms and related beliefs among two or more persons in the absence of an identifiable pathogen," implying that symptoms were "anxiety or stress induced."[36]

Moreover, the diagnosis had been applied exclusively to illness episodes among females—in girls' schools, women's clubs, and gender-segregated workplaces, especially among young women laboring on electronic assembly lines in Southeast Asia. Only in the 1990s was the diagnosis extended to men claiming Gulf War syndrome. An overview of published American cases of mass psychogenic illness by two NIOSH psychologists found that 93 percent of those diagnosed were women, describing this gendering as the diagnosis's "most obvious characteristic."[37] Peter Boxer, a University of Cincinnati doctor and professor of psychiatry, likewise saw the defining attribute in MPI cases as the presence of "relatively uneducated, low-paid women who perform highly routine tasks."[38] Michael Colligan, a NIOSH psychologist and promoter of the MPI diagnosis, was not unique in suggesting that the gendering of MPI was related to women's more "emotional nature," or to conflicts between work and family.[39] Other proponents went so far as to suggest that MPI was the result of that "uniquely feminine event, the menstrual cycle."[40] This tacit assertion was common in the pages of the *Journal for Occupational Medicine* during the 1960s, in which advertisements for tranquilizers targeted the treatment of pesky female patients unwilling to confess the menstrual nature of their problems. The advertisement for the diuretic and tranquilizer Cyclex—the very name of which invoked menstruation—recommended to doctors that they not depend on female patients to confess the true menstrual nature of their problems (Fig. 17). Such advertising made clear that women could not be trusted to report or even assess the true nature of their ill health. When it came to explaining the imperceptibility of a physical cause, the bodies laboring in office buildings became not simply human but female.

The diagnosis of MPI rarely sat easily with office workers. One promoter of the diagnosis observed that "individuals with psychogenic illnesses will often cling tenaciously to the idea that their illness is 'purely physical.'" This, however, did not stop him from applying the diagnosis in an incident when "not a single employee believed that psychological

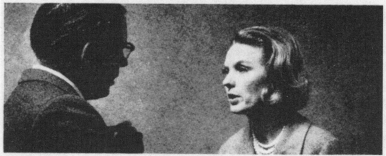

only a few women ever tell their doctors

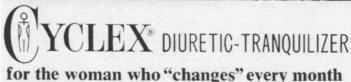

C̣YCLEX® DIURETIC-TRANQUILIZER

for the woman who "changes" every month

MSD MERCK SHARP & DOHME Division of Merck & Co., INC., West Point, Pa.

WHERE TODAY'S THEORY IS TOMORROW'S THERAPY

Figure 17. Pharmaceutical companies regularly promoted tranquilizers for female patients in the pages of the *Journal of Occupational Medicine*, often explicitly or implicitly suggesting that menstruation was at the root of women's complaints. In this 1965 advertisement, doctors are informed that they cannot trust what their female patients report because few will confess the true menstrual nature of their complaint. Notably, such advertisements often portrayed patients as white women in middle-class dress, invoking the tensions that emerged as middle-class women left the home for the workplace. At the same time, the racing and classing of this figure suggests that this medication was marketed for prescription to office workers.

factors played a significant role."[41] At work in the diagnosis of MPI was the not-so-veiled assumption that women were not trustworthy as registers of events in their own bodies. NIOSH psychologists held that "to the extent that the individual is able accurately to attribute existing discomforts to life and job-related stressors, susceptibility to mass psychogenic illness should decrease."[42] Cast as outside physical detection by a regime of apprehending chemical exposures materially embedded in the instruments and methods of industrial hygiene, office occupational health episodes were very often labeled as a troublesome pathology of perception misconnected to concrete matters of environment. Facing the failure of toxicology and aspersions of hysteria, what means were available to workers wanting to make claims about the presence and nature of chemical exposures in the twentieth century?

Popular Epidemiology and the Distribution of Conditions

Is your office too hot___ too cold___ drafty___ dusty___ other___?

Is the supply of air good___ inadequate___ no fresh air at all___?

Is the air circulation good___ poor___ no circulation at all___?

Are there irritating fumes in the air? yes___ no___

If yes, where do they come from?

—Office Workers Health and Safety Survey, 1981

I took out our health survey notebook and started to put squares and triangles and stars on a street map, with a different symbol for each disease group. . . . Suddenly a pattern emerged!—Gibbs, *Love Canal* (1982), 66–67

How might a worker have surmised that an errant molecule from this piece of carpet ended up in her lungs and was the specific irritant causing her headache, infection, or tumor? Toxicology, though a necessary proof for courtrooms, has not been the only widely practiced means of identifying hazardous environments. Surveys, like those conducted by the women office workers' movement, were an alternative method for materializing chemical exposures, not at the level of the individual but in the aggregates of community, neighborhood, or building. A tradition of surveys by nonscientists who have mapped degraded and unhealthful environments is at least a century old.

The sociologist Phil Brown coined the term *popular epidemiology* in 1987 to describe how working-class women like Lois Gibbs and Ann Anderson went from house to house surveying the incidence of family illnesses in their neighborhoods of Love Canal, New York, and Woburn, Massachusetts, in the 1970s.[43] Scholars have since named popular epidemiology as a cornerstone of contemporary community environmental activism.[44] Popular epidemiology is the practice by which laypeople, activists, and sympathetic scientists collect and organize empirical information to identify health problems in the place where they live or work. Also called commonsense, street-side, creek-side, or "housewife" epidemiology, it was responsible for the identification of most incidents of community toxic exposure and workplace cancer clusters in late-twentieth-century America.[45]

Crack open the popular epidemiology of the late twentieth century. It was composed of an assemblage of tools, practices, and subject positions quite different from toxicology. While toxicology captured and made sense of chemical exposures in laboratories, where scientists isolated a chemical's signature physiological effects under highly controlled experimental settings, popular epidemiology, in contrast, took place in the field, where local people mapped the *distribution* of a health problem and its spatial proximity to industry and related plumes or odors. While toxicology objectified specific chemicals, popular epidemiology mapped health onto the social and spatial distribution of difference in the built environment. While toxicology held bodies to be predictable and universalizable, popular epidemiology allowed bodies to be diverse in their reaction to a common environment.

The women office workers' movement followed in toxic-waste activists' footsteps when it began using surveys to collect wide-ranging health complaints in office buildings in the early 1980s. The elements of this assemblage, however, originated in the social survey movement of the Progressive Era. Social surveys were a tradition of descriptive data collection by activists, settlements, marginal social scientists, and charities first practiced in the 1880s, before the discipline of sociology was established in American universities.[46] The first social surveys in the United States originated with settlement houses that stressed the role of knowledge in social reform work. Knowledge came through two activities: the personal experience of living amid a poor community and empirical, intimate, house-by-house investigations. Residence in a settlement was believed to foster empathy; a reformer was "to be as a neighbor among neighbors; to hear day by day the stolid, terrible gossip of the street; to take, as one insensibly comes to take, the point of view on matters moral and physical of people sleeping seven in a room."[47] While living amid the working class and poor whom they sought to serve through good works, settlement house reformers "Americanized" new immigrants, provided classes in literacy, art, and cooking and supplied day care, recreation, and public health services to local families. Inspired by Charles Booth's survey, *Life and Labor in London* (1899–1903), the American social survey movement practiced firsthand investigation of the conditions of a community in order to formulate programs of amelioration, sharing a positivist faith in science's ability to bring about social change.

W. E. B. DuBois's *The Philadelphia Negro* (1899), inspired by Booth's study, was one of the first social surveys published in America.[48] Financed by the Quaker Philadelphia Settlement, the study set out to "lay before the public such a body of information" as to point to a solution for the "Negro Problem" in the seventh ward.[49] Typical of social surveyors who would follow, DuBois and his assistants went house to house with a series of schedules interviewing residents on everything from where they lived to their education, occupations, health, criminality, pauperism, socializing, and family life. The third of six schedules used surveyed "the environment of the Negro," asking questions about housing, crowding, yards, sanitation, water closets, windows, washing, ventilation, light, and cleanliness. The results were ordered in detailed chapters, simple quantitative charts, and house-scale maps (see Fig. 18). As the historian Mia Bay has argued, DuBois undertook *The Philadelphia Negro* as a deliberate departure from the research methods used by both black and white scholars of race.[50] By assembling empirical evidence, DuBois moved away from assertions of natural laws explaining race, and away from seeing blacks as a single, undifferentiable mass. DuBois's study sought "to extract from a complicated mass of facts the tangible evidence of social atmosphere surrounding Negroes, which differs from that surrounding most whites."[51] The purpose was to document a "social condition and environment" instead of a biological racial one.[52] DuBois's survey had two qualities typical of social surveys: first, a multiplicity or diversity of aggregated expressions and, second, "conditions" rather than discrete causes.

UNIVERSITY OF PENNSYLVANIA.

CONDITION OF THE NEGROES OF PHILADELPHIA, WARD SEVEN.

Home Schedule, 3.

DECEMBER 1, 1896.   No.————————   Investigator.

1 Material of house? . . . .
2 Stories in house above basement ? . . . .
3 Number of homes in house? . . . .
4 In which story is this home ? . . . .
5 Number of rooms in this home ? . . . . . .
6 Is this home rented directly of the landlord ? . . . . .
7 Number of boarders in this home ? . . . . .
8 Number of lodgers in this home ? . . . .
9 Number of servants kept? . . . .
10 Total number of persons in this home ? . . . .
11 House owned by . . . .
12 Rent paid monthly? . . . . .
13 Rent received from sub-letting ? . . . .
14 Bath-room ? . . . .
15 Water-closet ? . . . .
16 Privy ? . . . .
17 Yard, and size ? . . . .
18 Where is washing hung to dry ? . . . .
19 Light ? . . . .
20 Ventilation and air ? . . . .
21 Cleanliness ? . . . .
22 Outside sanitary conditions ? . . . .

THE HOME.

		Room No. 1.	Room No. 2.	Room No. 3.	Room No. 4.	Room No. 5.	Room No. 6.
23	Use ?						
24	Dimensions ?						
25	Outside windows ?						
26	Furniture ?						
27	Occupants at night ?						
28	Additional rooms ?						

29 When and where have you had difficulty in renting houses?

Figure 18. This schedule for a survey of home environments was developed and used by DuBois in his study of Negroes in Philadelphia's seventh ward. Results from the schedules were often tallied in straightforward tables. In addition, the distribution of the "Negro inhabitants" and their economic status were plotted on a large fold-out color map. DuBois, *Philadelphia Negro.*

Most settlement houses in the East, however, had a poorer record of dealing with racial difference, excluding blacks, holding segregated activities, or simply locating themselves in white-majority neighborhoods.[53] Settlements typically served as important opportunities for white middle-class women who had attained greater access but still lacked prospects for professional employment. Jane Addams's Hull House, the most famous of the settlement houses and the one of which Alice Hamilton was a member, also produced a well-respected social survey, *The Hull-House Maps and Papers* (1895). Florence Kelley, who researched child labor for the survey, became the first female factory inspector in Illinois and later director of the National Consumer League. She argued that such social science undertakings were especially suited to women who brought "humane" concerns to their endeavor.[54] Like DuBois, Hull House women armed with paper and pencils recorded detailed information in house-to-house interviews with schedules: "The manner of investigation has been painstaking, and the facts set forth are as trustworthy as personal inquiry and intelligent effort could make them. Not only was each house, tenement, and room visited and inspected, but in many cases the reports obtained from one person were corroborated by many others, and statements from different workers at the same trades and occupations, as to wages and unemployed seasons, served as mutual confirmation."[55] The merits and truthfulness of the survey, so they argued, came from its attention to excruciating particulars, a "greater minuteness" that gave the research "a photographic reproduction of Chicago's poorest quarters."[56] Like other social surveys, Hull House research paid careful attention to and wrote vibrant descriptions of the built environments of both life and labor. "Little idea," testified the introduction to a middle-class readership, "can be given of the filthy rooms and rotten tenements, the dingy courts and tumble-down sheds, the foul stables and dilapidated outhouses, the broken sewer pipes, the piles of garbage fairly alive with diseased odors."[57] Through prose, simple statistics, and colorful maps, surveys provided testimony meant to move the middle-class public to reform and the state to intervention. Progressive Era women reformers successfully used social surveys to gain the passage of legislation concerning lead in the workplace and child labor.

The subject position investigators fashioned in the practice of social surveys differed markedly from the detached and apolitical stance of university toxicologists and industrial hygienists. Requiring investigators to live in the communities they studied, social surveys expressed a "geographic sentiment" that sought to describe empathetically local conditions.[58] According to Florence Kelley, you must "suffer from the dirty streets, the universal ugliness, the lack of oxygen in the air you breathe, the endless struggle with soot and dust and insufficient water supply . . . if you are to speak as one having authority and not as the scribes in these matters of common daily life and experience."[59] Likewise, DuBois sought to study the seventh ward "personally and not by proxy" with "not lack of human interest and moral conviction, but rather the heart-quality of fairness."[60] While Hull House women used empathetic eyes to observe neighbors whom they nonetheless understood as different from themselves, DuBois conducted his social science research into the "Negro Problem" with a keen sense of himself as also a black man. His observations were recorded through a "double-consciousness, this sense of always looking at one's self through the eyes of others, of measuring one's soul by the tape of a world that looks on in amused contempt and pity."[61] Moreover, observers were typically multiple. While employing a single schedule, social surveys usually required multiple door-to-door interviewers who gathered information from as many people as lived in the neighborhood. Social surveys, thus, did not represent themselves as providing a representative or universalizable view but a comprehensive and empathetic realism, captured through an aggregate of multiple prisms that mapped the distribution and diversity of conditions in a highly localized community.

The most extensive social survey was the six-volume Pittsburgh Survey of 1906–7, which was undertaken as part of the charity movement.[62] Funded by the Russell Sage Foundation, the survey was conducted by some of the community's middle-class members as a self-study and exhibited to the public as a means to solve social problems. The Department of Surveys and Exhibits at the Russell Sage Foundation, as well as local civic bodies, funded thousands of such surveys through the 1940s. The movement reached its peak in the late 1920s; 2,775 surveys were published in 1927 alone.[63] Social surveys expressed a reformist science tradition, but also an understanding of science as open to amateurs and attached to, rather than detached from, communities. With the establishment of academic sociology and the rise of the sample survey for marketing and polling, the social survey movement dwindled in the years before the Second World War.[64]

It was only after the Second World War, however, that American epidemiologists began to use complex statistical methods to rigorously and analytically calculate the relative risks of specific behaviors or factors for chronic illnesses. With the recent advent of antibiotics and the hard-won gains of sanitation reform, the demographics of sickness in twentieth-century America had shifted from the killer infectious diseases that terrorized nineteenth-century life. Cancer and heart disease were now, if not more prevalent, at least more visible dangers. Large epidemiological studies contended with physiologist experimentalists to find the causes of heart disease and lung cancer. Professional epidemiological studies increasingly created, and not just found, their data sets with diagnostic tools like X-rays, spirometers, and blood-cell counts that required expertise and technical facilities to interpret. With large samples and controls, such studies could make strong probabilistic predictions. By the 1970s, heart disease was linked to high-fat diets and lung cancer to cigarette smoking. Habits and substances that had been habitually, unproblematically, and even pleasurably part of daily life were marked as dangerous.

Linking behaviors with diseases depended on educating the public in epidemiological logic. Through public education campaigns, the "new public health" sought not only to persuade ordinary people to change their behaviors but also to interiorize a popular version of the risk calculus.[65] Good citizens were to evaluate their own behaviors and lifestyles not simply on moral grounds but also according to a risk analysis aided by popularized epidemiological findings. Dangers could be found in daily life.

Once perceived, the connection between industrial chemicals and health could not be confined to the factory floor, the corporate laboratory, or professional scientific circles. Workers went home after work and noticed that their houses lay under the plume of the factory that employed them, or that effluent was habitually dumped into the ditch around the corner, or that the new synthetic materials they consumed and which surrounded them were manufactured out of the same potentially hazardous chemicals. After decades of affluent commodity culture, the hazards of chemicals seeped out of factories and into the messy American imaginary. The chemical presence that industrialization had produced and which had "streamed" into everyday life, in Rachel Carson's words, cast "a shadow that is no less ominous because it is formless and obscure."[66] The difficulty of perceiving formless and obscure chemical exposures did not make them any less present or frightening to the public.

Though it was in a certain sense made possible by a popularized risk calculus, popular epidemiology offered an alternative to the extremely targeted and technical format of medical studies. The tools and practices of popular epidemiology were cheaply and readily available in daily life: a pencil, the telephone, notebooks, newspaper ads, church meetings, door-to-door canvassing, photocopy machines, and published maps. While it would be wrong to say that popular epidemiologists were opposed to using diagnostic tests, their method of collecting intimate and anecdotal knowledge through house-by-house canvassing involved an implicit critique of the narrowly technical and impersonal studies that dominated scientific investigations and debates. Popular epidemiologists were not against science but *for* accessible knowledge and community involvement.

Working-class and low-income women, not middle-class reformers, have been overwhelmingly the main practitioners of popular epidemiology. As frequent targets of public health campaigns and long-standing subjects of middle-class charity, working-class communities had encountered opportunities to watch science in action and develop a critical assessment of public health and state- or industry-sponsored science. Working-class women of the 1970s built on and transformed the intimate and geographical standpoint of the social survey—they were simultaneously the subjects of their investigations and the investigators. Moreover, they were much more skeptical of science than the social surveyors had been, and, like so many during the 1970s, they were suspicious of expertise. The critical perspective from which popular epidemiologists saw regulatory science in action was not, however, an antiscience stance but the performance of a counterexpertise.[67] For popular epidemiologists, science was not an apolitical arbiter but a tool that both sides of a struggle could use.

As self-fashioned experts in science, working-class women extended the swell of labor activism to the home and responded to the hail of a renewed feminism. Working-class white women, in particular, were the first to establish self-help groups and feminist women's health clinics, which encouraged women to take medicine in their own hands through vaginal self-exam, menstrual extraction, and participatory health clinics.[68] Popular epidemiology was yet another example of working-class women fashioning themselves as counterexperts entitled to use science (the results of one of their neighborhood surveys are mapped in Fig. 19). However, the women who found themselves gathering neighborhood surveys were rarely motivated as feminists; more typically they were mothers who had become activists on behalf of their children, carrying on the tradition of maternalist reformism.[69] In this way, popular epidemiologists both drew on and subverted gender roles by becoming community leaders and spokespersons in the name of motherhood. Though toxic-waste activists did not organize *as* women, the Citizens Clearinghouse for Hazardous Waste, an organization founded by Lois Gibbs in 1981 to provide guidance to newly minted community activists, recognized that women were the primary actors. Among their many training manuals, including one on how to conduct a community health survey, they published a pamphlet titled *Empowering Ourselves: Women and Toxic Organizing* (1989), which gave advice on the gender politics of activism.[70] The manual discussed the paradox of organizing as mothers: in daily-life terms, activism meant spending less time with one's family, which could lead to marital strife, divorce, or even physical abuse by a fed-up spouse. Both popular epidemiology activists and their opponents were keenly aware of the political work gendered activism could do: calling on motherhood could marshal a tradition of protectionism and justify bringing emotion into deliberations, while at the same time it provided a wedge by which opponents could illegitimate activists' expertise and voices, accusing them of being "hysterical housewives."[71]

The intimate and geographical methods of data collection that popular epidemiologists crafted drew on already gendered practices. As mothers, socially charged with the care of family health, community women were the informants and organizers of popular epidemiology. Women who stayed home to take care of small children had opportunities to become intimately aware of the changes their neighborhood had undergone over long stretches of time. They might remember changes in the odor of the air or the taste of water, or in their yards and pets; they might have witnessed the illegal dumping of waste far in the past, or they or their husbands might have worked at the neighborhood factory under suspicion. Popular epidemiologists were expansive in the kinds of information

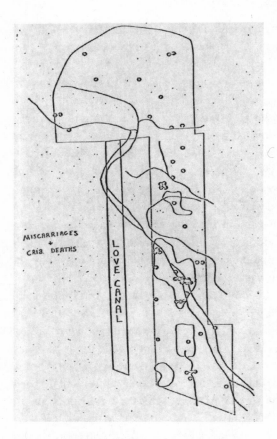

Figure 19. Hand-drawn map of miscarriages and crib deaths, based on a house-to-house survey by Lois Gibbs of the Love Canal Homeowners Association, and a local geneticist, Beverley Paigen. Other maps plotted birth defects, nervous breakdowns, and urinary disease. These maps, largely based on information provided by mothers on the health of their families, were used to argue that health effects converged along water routes or swales that connected more distant homes to the toxic-waste dumping site. Beverley Paigen, "Health Hazards at Love Canal," testimony before the House Subcommittee on Oversight and Investigations, March 21, 1979. Love Canal Collection, University Archives, State University of New York at Buffalo. Courtesy of Beverly Paigen.

they gathered, recording a variety of illnesses and symptoms, from rashes to learning disabilities to cancer. Photocopied surveys typically included "other" and provided space for informants to elaborate. Their conversations with neighbors might also include topics such as city politics or the disposition of the local physician. They were not restricted to enumerating illnesses and instead often gathered highly personal anecdotes of failed gardens in backyards, smelly moisture in the basement, frequent trips to doctors, confusing and conflicting diagnoses, as well as the stress of uncertainty. The anecdotal mode provided room for emotion and individual life stories to become part of the analysis. Penny Newman, a well-known toxic-waste activist, eloquently described how evidence was based on intimate experience: "While others gather their information from textbooks and reports, we live, breathe and die this issue. . . . We're the ones that have watched as our communities have become devastated; we've seen homes disappear. We're the ones that must lie awake listening to our children struggle to breathe; who comfort the young woman who has suffered her 6th miscarriage. . . . Yes, we know the issue better than anyone."[72] Observations came from gendered, classed, and often explicitly raced social locations that incorporated, rather than excluded, subjective, and emotional knowledge.

For white toxic-waste activists of the late 1970s and the 1980s, especially homeowners like those in the Love Canal Homeowners' Association, observations were likely grounded in outrage over unexpected violations of their families' personal safety. At Love Canal, homeowners came to realize that the grassy park in the center of their neighborhood capped a decades-old toxic-waste site.[73] Feelings of entitlement to safety came from expectations rooted, not in a subordinate class status, but in white privilege.[74] Pollution materially expressed a tension between expectation and actuality.

In polluted communities with many African Americans near incinerators or factories, such as the chemical and petrochemical manufacturing corridors of Louisiana, Texas, and New Jersey, residents daily witnessed the movement of pollution from factory to neighborhood with their eyes and other senses.[75] Women in some long-standing working-class neighborhoods were already members of established benevolent societies or women's clubs, such as the Newtown Florist club, organized earlier in the century to collect money to cover the regular funerals and sickness associated with their industrialized neighborhood, or even to agitate for

better municipal services.[76] African-American environmental activists
tended to ground their analysis in terms of social justice and infringe-
ments of civil rights, articulating the fight to live in healthy environments
as akin to struggles for better schools, municipal services, and housing.
For African-American communities in Louisiana's "cancer alley," for
example, residents connected the distribution of pollution with historically rooted structural inequalities.[77] Some of the first analyses of "environmental racism" used zip codes and government demographic data
on the race of residents to map out the parallel between distributions of
incinerators and dumps and the locations of poor neighborhoods of
color.[78] Like DuBois in The Philadelphia Negro, studies of environmental
racism emphasized the historical origins of injustice. Thus the intimate
and proximate view of community health surveys was used to demonstrate either unfulfilled privilege or historically sedimented injustices.

Intimate and geographical reasoning could be a powerful counter-
weight to statistical and toxicological reasoning. If an industry representative claimed that a chemical posed only a one in ten thousand chance
of causing fatalities, an activist could reframe the risk assessment as
asserting that it is acceptable for one person in the neighborhood, perhaps a child, to die.[79] Or if an expert claimed that a chemical exposure
did not exceed its threshold limit value, an activist could retort that
children, pregnant women, and elderly people in the neighborhood
lived under a plume twenty-four hours a day, seven days a week, and not
just between nine and five in a controlled factory setting.[80] While toxicology traced the effects of chemicals in stimuli-reduced experimental settings, popular epidemiology mapped human relationships in a muddy,
unrestrained, lived place. The assemblage of tools, practices, and subject
positions that structured popular epidemiology made perceptible, not
specific causal pathways, but the spatial distribution of inequalities and
tensions of place.

By the time the women office workers' movement began encouraging
popular epidemiology surveys of buildings in the early 1980s, a range of
practical assistance and manuals were available for the beginning popular epidemiologist.[81] Lois Gibbs's Citizens Clearinghouse for Hazardous
Waste, later renamed the Center for Health, Environment, and Justice,
was only the biggest of many nonprofit organizations teaching and
using popular epidemiology. While not institutionalized in the same

way as toxicology or industrial hygiene, popular epidemiology became firmly sedimented in the practices of grassroots environmentalism.

Popular epidemiology mapped health effects onto the physical presence of factories, dumps, incinerators, or even manufactured products. Mapping evoked a chemical exposure's proximate and diverse conditions rather than its specific dimensions. Instead of pinpointing the precise chemical cause and predictable physiological response, place-based surveys, first, fashioned an aggregate health problem out of an array of particularized experiences and, second, mapped a collectivity of health effects onto a concurring social inequality or tension of place. Surveys were able to situate a problem in its location and not in the individual. A popular epidemiology study could conclude that "in this neighborhood, along the old creeks, by these factories, many people suffer from rashes and respiratory illnesses," or "in this office building, in the offices with unopenable windows and new carpet, many workers have health complaints," or "toxic dumps are located in these neighborhoods, where low-income African Americans live, where there is a high prevalence of asthma."

Thus popular epidemiology generated its own domain of imperceptibility. Concurrence, not cause, was apprehended, leaving uncertainty still at the center of responses to low-level chemical exposures. Spatial and intimate reasoning, however, was not without its own persuasiveness. For nonexperts, maps were more accessible than statistics and thus useful for publicizing a health problem. As a result, one of the foremost goals of popular epidemiology was to instigate an EPA, public health, or NIOSH investigation. Popular epidemiology did not do a better job than toxicology at identifying a molecular culprit; rather, it was a more powerful technique for apprehending aggregates of nonspecific health effects caused by nonacute exposures in the messy world of people's lives, if not in the empty box of the lab.

Existence in the Encounter

Industrial hygiene and popular epidemiology collided both in polluted neighborhoods and in office buildings. Sick building syndrome came into existence as a phenomenon lodged in this encounter. Sick building syndrome's strange shape was traced out by what each could and could not perceive about the nature of environmental health.

As previous chapters have shown, office buildings were constructed as places where comfort and efficiency could be delivered mechanically. When the office's veneer of middle-class ambiance began to slip, workers' burgeoning apprehension of office work as oppressive in its details was confronted with a built environment designed to deliver comfort. In turn, deviations from comfort, which industrial workers would have accepted with a shrug, became bodily signals of oppression. With easy access to paper, pencil, and photocopier, office workers used popular epidemiology methods to assemble these multitudes of health complaints into a buildingwide health event. The office building's walls became the phenomenon's bounds, and the shifting field of symptoms was its expression. This phenomenon, now formed by its very collection of difference, was confronted with instruments and methods from industrial hygiene that required toxic exposures to be both regular and specific, in turn rendering ubiquitous and low-level exposures unprovable and imperceptible. Sick building syndrome became a phenomenon characterized as much by what could not be perceived—specific cause— as by what could be. It became a phenomenon whose very existence contained uncertainty, multiplicity, and nonspecificity.

The strange shape of sick building syndrome made it a difficult problem to assert. While some thought sBs was nothing more than mass psychogenic illness and others that a specific cause would someday be found, sBs was technically defined in a way that held in negotiation two very different regimes of perceptibility, two different ontologies of exposure. sBs was a phenomenon of expression only: an "occurrence of an excessive number of subjective complaints by the occupants of a building."[82] The EPA's definition underlined its acausal form, demarcating sBs as "a set of symptoms that affect some number of building occupants during the time they spend in the building. It cannot be traced to specific pollutants or sources within the building."[83] To underscore this nonspecific definition, another term, *building-related illness*, was used to describe cases in which a specific cause was found, such as in cases of Legionnaires' disease or asbestos contamination. In short, if a cause was found, a building no longer had sick building syndrome. Sick building syndrome's odd definition encompassed nonspecificity both in cause (as nonspecific pollution as defined by toxicology) and in effect (as diverse symptom experiences as captured by popular epidemiology). We can see this uneasy meeting of ontologies in the following explanation of sBS, written by two university researchers in the mid-1980s:

> Because there is not an all-embracing and comprehensive definition of the term, sick building syndrome has been viewed with some skepticism; however, one need only interview workers from an air conditioned building for a short time before becoming aware of the frequency of symptoms experienced by them. The cause is not known, the symptoms are non-specific, there is nothing abnormal to measure, and there is no laboratory challenge test to reproduce the symptoms. Therefore a definition in the usual scientific terms is not possible.[84]

In other words, sick building syndrome was the name for a phenomenon materialized by the contentious encounter of two different but nonetheless effective and truth-telling ways of materializing chemical exposures.

Perhaps partially because it came to exist in this encounter instead of being the product of a single secure discipline, the unconventional qualities that the name *sick building syndrome* made sense of sparked an intense, though simplistic, debate formulated in all-or-nothing terms: Is sick building syndrome a real, physically caused, phenomenon or not? Any historical research on sick building syndrome is necessarily an intervention into this tense terrain, not least because of the ongoing struggles of people to demonstrate the effects of chemical exposure on their lives. The politics of chemical exposure, whether in streams, offices, or neighborhoods is caught in a tangle of multiple histories. Each of these histories populates the world with different kinds of relationships and imbues exposures with divergent qualities, while at the same time producing domains of imperceptibility. These domains of imperceptibility fundamentally shape phenomena, and charting them can help us to navigate uncertainty. Seen in this light, the terms of the question "real or not?" are profoundly inadequate. Uncertainty was not a quality to be resolved, but the nature of exposure.

Scientists, too, were caught between these conflicting ways of knowing and inhabiting the world. They themselves worked in office buildings and knew all too well the limits of sanctioned methods. While this chapter has emphasized the best practices of industrial hygienists, toxicologists, and popular epidemiologists, the actual deployment of techniques and experiments were undertaken in a political and even unethical terrain of corporate science, antiregulation, and racialized environmental injustice. Government scientists, in particular, had to navigate hostile administrations, racially segregated landscapes and workplaces, and corporate rebuttals to make positive claims about chemical exposures. Imperceptibility, as the next chapter will argue, was not just about what a method or discipline could not do. Imperceptibility was a result actively sought and produced so that chemical exposures could become something which no one could do anything about.

Uncertainty, Race, and Activism at the EPA

These things happen to people in poor areas. Society is set up in such a way that it is the poor and the uneducated who suffer the main impact of natural and man-made disasters. People in low-lying areas get the floods, people in shanties get the hurricanes and tornadoes. . . . I'm not just a college professor, I'm a head of a department. I don't see myself fleeing an airborne toxic event.—Jack Gladney in DeLillo, *White Noise*, 114–17

[5] **What happens when chemical** exposures do not obey systems of privilege? Society is set up to protect the privileged from toxic events, or so the neurotic protagonist of the novel *White Noise* insists. In the novel, Gladney's affluence produces both anxiety and blindness about his vulnerability to errant plumes and accidental spills. When a toxic cloud from a train accident floats over his suburban neighborhood, Gladney finds himself on the run despite his worldly advantages. Even systems of privilege can disappoint.

"White noise" is a technical term describing a steady complex unobtrusive sound, such as the drone of a fan, that drowns out, or makes imperceptible, other surrounding sounds. As a metaphor, white noise suggests that imperception can be generated. Perception is characterized by historically specific modes of paying attention, which always necessitated strategic suspensions of perception.[1] Perception involves historically produced disengagements from a broader field of bombardments for the sake of concentrating on and rendering intelligible a more narrowly differentiated set of phenomena. In other words, focusing on a single signal entails a learned inattention to other noise. These suspensions of perception, moreover, result not just in passive disengagements but also the production of historically specific terrains of invisibility, the outcome of what I am calling regimes of perceptibility.

This chapter explores imperceptibility and its relation to chemical

exposures and race through a case study of activism by government
scientists in the U.S. Environmental Protection Agency, the federal
agency charged with investigating chemical exposures and setting national standards. Even more narrowly, I will focus on one idiosyncratic
event at the EPA: the political activism of EPA scientists organized around
an incident of chemical exposure at the agency's own Washington, D.C.,
headquarters in the 1980s. Through workplace activism and unionization, these scientists sought to resist the production of uncertainty and
imperceptibility generated at the nexus of state, corporate, scientific, and
juridical practices. At the same time that the EPA was developing national
standards and embroiled in questions of scientific uncertainty, it was also
shaped by local racialized geographies of the particular neighborhood in
which its offices stood.

In the late-twentieth-century United States, both critics of and apolo-
gists for racism typically saw it as an issue concerning the disadvantag-
ing of people with marked racialized identities, often called "visible
minorities," emphasizing the role of perception in defining difference.
Scholarly attention to relationships between racism and science, including environmental issues, has followed this same pattern. Historians of
science have tended to take up questions of race only when examining
acts of racism or when "race" has been the subject of science. Much less
attention has been paid to the inverse subject of racialized disadvantage
—the work of racialized privilege.[2] Furthermore, virtually no attention
has been paid to the work of racialization in scientific practices not
explicitly about race, in practices we could call normal science. One of
the reasons this gap persists is that racialized privilege itself has often
operated through its invisibility to those who possess it, and thus has
rarely been named as such.[3] It is difficult to research the work of race
when historical actors did not mark it themselves.

In contrast to the early twentieth century, when those who benefited
from and upheld white supremacy explicitly and frequently named and
invoked it, the desegregating cold war era produced a liberalism that
provided a newly articulated and powerful refashioning of "race" as a
social, rather than biological, phenomenon. Racism was increasingly
defined as an individually held psychological prejudice that prevented
the ideal colorless meritocracy from emerging. Race was thus an artifact
of color vision. In turn, whiteness could be held as an unraced identity;
its very colorlessness fostered a belief among those who enjoyed it in the

possibility of a better "color-blind" society.[4] By the 1980s, the colorless location of "whiteness" and the confinement of racism to the realm of the psychological encouraged white U.S. citizens to suspend their awareness of persistent racialized distributions of privilege and to look only for expressions of racialized disadvantage. White privilege operated through this regularized suspension of perception—in other words, through a regime of imperception. Instead of government-sanctioned signs over water fountains and doorways, in the late twentieth century white privilege was generated, like white noise, precisely by "seeming not to be anything in particular."[5]

This chapter seeks to explore the inverse of how U.S. communities of color theorized race in their development of environmental justice—that is, how the practice and activism of predominantly white, professional-class state environmental scientists in the 1980s were shaped by the racialized location of their work and lives. I use the term *racialization* to underscore that "race" was not a possession of persons prior to social arrangements of power but rather was produced by those arrangements. Likewise, individuals did not own privilege. They enacted and generated it both intentionally and unintentionally through pervasive racialization. Instead of asking whether individual scientists held racist views, this chapter tries to understand how scientists' various political and scientific positions were shaped by the racialized world in which they lived. The science at the EPA was not racist science; it was not concerned with defining racial kinds or measuring superiority or inferiority. Instead, science at the EPA was normal science, and as such took place in the unfortunately unexceptional racialized circumstances of the United States. Thus this chapter takes up the difficult task of connecting two different, yet coexisting, regimes of imperceptibility in late-twentieth-century America: first, the uncertainty of chemical exposures and, second, the unmarked location of racialized privilege.

Racing and Placing the EPA

The physical condition and location of the EPA's headquarters, in south-west Washington's Waterside Mall, was symbolic of both the inequalities within the capital and the agency's neglect and low standing under the Reagan Administration. An ugly, beige, concrete and glass complex built in 1970 stood on land cleared in one of the federal government's biggest urban renewal programs. Previously, the Southwest neighborhood had been notorious for its alleyway slums, in which the city's poorest black residents were crowded together by a segregated housing market.[6] The bulldozing and redevelopment of the area displaced more than ten thousand African-American "alley dwellers."[7] In place of low-income housing came a shopping mall called Waterside, flanked by two twelve-story towers of upscale apartments. When, in an era of white flight from city centers, the apartment towers failed to attract renters, the real estate developer leased his building to the federal government, which in turned assigned it in 1971 to the newly founded EPA.

The presence of the EPA headquarters in this downtown area was part of the more general schizophrenic character of Washington, D.C., a finely segregated Southern city profoundly shaped in terms of "black" and "white." Yet serving as the nation's capital, it was also a meeting place for the North and the South, as well as for the national and the local.[8] In the EPA's Southwest neighborhood, located within walking distance of the National Mall, grand government agencies and luxury apartments sat uneasily next to public housing and racialized unemployment and homelessness. Waterside was just a ten-minute drive from the site of one of the most violent riots that followed Martin Luther King Jr.'s assassination, two years prior to Waterside's construction. It was a neighborhood to which many of the poor residents of Southwest alleys had been displaced, some of whom lost their neighborhood yet again in the riot's flames.[9] Nonetheless segregation in the city was imperfect; by 1989, a few years after the chemical exposure event I will examine in this chapter, African Americans from a wide spectrum of classes made up 61 percent of the Southwest neighborhood's residents, while European Americans made up 35 percent.[10] Racialized spaces were minutely distributed within neighborhoods, buildings, and workplaces as much as between them.

The racialized geography of Washington, D.C., exemplified the persistence of geographical distributions of privilege that, as scholar George Lipsitz has argued, characterized the cold war era of government-mandated *desegregation*.[11] For example, large corporations accommodated state desegregation orders by channeling recently hired African Americans into racially segregated departments that relied on devalued technologies and skills.[12] Suburbanization and middle-class "white flight" during desegregation led to 4 million whites' moving out of city centers, while the number of whites living in suburbs increased by 22 million from 1966 to 1977.[13] Access to mortgages, loans, municipal services, and other government-sponsored privileges became correspondingly concentrated in the suburbs.[14] By 1993, the results of white flight meant that 80 percent of the nation's suburban whites lived in places with a black population under 1 percent.[15] In the Washington metropolitan area, 90.3 percent of European Americans lived in the suburbs, helping to make African Americans the vast majority of metropolitan residents. African Americans constituted 71.1 percent of the District's residents but only 8.2 percent of the population in its suburbs.[16]

Such patterns of desegregation also extended to workplaces of the federal government, which since passage of the Civil Rights Act of 1964 had hired large numbers of local African Americans to work in its bureaucracies. In the EPA headquarters and Waterside Mall, if not in their home neighborhoods, predominantly white scientists and professionals interacted daily with African Americans: in the shopping mall with African-American customers, sales clerks, and cleaning staff, and in the EPA itself with African-American secretaries, administrative assistants, and security personnel—and a few African-American professionals. The passage from the shopping mall into the headquarters marked a boundary between local and national spaces as well as between majority African-American and majority European-American spaces. While the EPA has not published longitudinal data, in 2001 black workers made up over half of the clerical staff at the agency's headquarters but only 8.2 percent of the professional-class workforce, of which whites composed 81.5 percent.[17] It is also useful to look at the racialization of "grade levels," the system by which seniority and pay is ranked in federal bureaucracies. While white workers made up 87.9 percent of the highest rank, GS15, and only 21.8 percent of the lowest ranks, GS14, black workers composed 65.4 percent of workers in the ranks below GS4 and only a sliver, 6.8 percent, of the highest rank.[18]

While the EPA was physically situated in a particular neighborhood, its charge was to establish regulations and standards for the whole nation. By the 1980s, most people saw the agency as failing in its mission. A multitude of reasons explained why so many EPA investigators were thwarted in their efforts to make strong claims about the health effects of chemical exposures. For one, exposures themselves were often transient and complicated. For another, sometimes the failure was a product of the difficulty and uncertainty plaguing good faith efforts to meet narrow juridical standards, which asked scientists to find causality in an individual chemical signal separated from the white noise of the built environment. At other times, the failure was a product of the EPA's methods and instruments, which had been designed to detect straightforward exposures in factory settings and not chronic or transient exposures in neighborhoods and offices. Thus a terrain of imperceptibility was hardwired into the very instruments investigators used. However, failure could also result from their position as government scientists, tightly restricted in their ability to communicate findings or design studies by politically appointed administrators whose ideology often rejected the notion that the state should regulate capitalism. EPA scientists were awkwardly positioned as civil servants accountable to the citizens, the state, and corporations, on the one hand, and as scientific spokespersons for "nature" and truth, on the other.

Since the 1980 televised struggle at Love Canal that culminated sensationally in two EPA agents' being taken hostage by community women, EPA scientists have become the regular villains in all too common dramas around chemical exposures. This plotline has agency investigators arriving at the instigation of local community activism, and then failing to come up with evidence useful to or commensurate with residents' accounts. As sociologist Celene Krauss argues, the white working-class communities, especially women, who protested against toxic waste in the 1970s and early 1980s saw their problems as tied to the failure of government-sponsored protections.[19] Lois Gibbs, an influential toxic-waste activist who got her start at Love Canal, described her investment in the government this way: "I grew up in a blue-collar community, it was very patriotic, into democracy. . . . I believed in government. . . . I believed that if you had a complaint, you went to the right person in the government. If there was a way to solve the problem, they would be glad to do it."[20] It was when the state, often the EPA, failed to provide expected aid that women such as Gibbs first became politicized as activists. The ill repute with which EPA scientists contended was reflected in the advice activists gave one another about government investigations: "The government studies are also bogus. We just have to start out knowing that the Centers for Disease Control, the EPA, or any of these regulatory agencies are not telling the truth. When they come your way, tell them to go away. Tell them, 'We don't need your studies.' You don't need their studies, because then you are countering more than you were before they got there."[21] For many grassroots activists, as well as environmental journalists, the agency was simply not trustworthy. In a short time, the EPA had flipped in many eyes from optimistic offshoot of Earth Day to obstructer of environmental justice.

During the 1980s, this already unsatisfying situation turned worse; EPA scientists went from frustrated to obstructed. When Republican candidate Ronald Reagan was elected president, he was forthright about his antienvironmentalist, proindustry, deregulation positions. The EPA —just ten years old when Reagan began his first term—had been founded in a reformist moment when the expansion of the state was greeted with liberal optimism, guided by a "progressive" and technocratic conviction that objective, scientific expertise would solve problems of the social and natural orders. Many of the scientists hired then believed that their science could improve the nation if not the world.[22] The 1980s, however, were a time of backlash against state regulation, believed to hinder economic progress, and EPA scientists saw their position as trustworthy and privileged experts expire. Reagan proposed a 60 percent cut in the EPA's budget and a 40 percent cut in staff.[23] Though the Democratic-controlled Congress put up some resistance, most cuts went through and the administrative staff was overhauled.

Most detrimental was the appointment of Ann Gorsuch (1981–83) as head of the EPA. Gorsuch filled the agency's upper administrative ranks with professionals who had made their living defending industry against regulation. Rather than acting as a conservative steward, she set out to declaw the agency, stripping it of its regulatory capacity in practice if not in rule.[24] Gorsuch, nicknamed the "Ice Queen" within the agency, tacked up a brightly colored "hit list" in her office, which indicated career staff targeted for dismissal.[25] Scientists who resisted pressure to repress damning data or acted as whistle-blowers could find themselves fired, harassed, or transferred to positions in which their only tasks would be answering phones or filing papers. Reagan made Gorsuch's job easier by signing a series of executive orders that prevented the EPA from collecting information about a chemical for possible regulation without the sanction of the Office of Management and Budget (OMB). OMB only gave its approval if the cost-benefit analysis it ran proved to be economical for industries. The regulatory process could now be stopped before it even began, placing economic considerations squarely before those of science. Gorsuch was followed by William Ruckelshaus (1983–85), who left his position at the timber company Weyerhaeuser, a frequent target of environmentalist groups. Next came Lee Thomas (1985–89), who afterward became senior vice president at the pulp and paper company Georgia-Pacific. At its nadir in the 1980s, the regulatory agency was being run, with little pretense at neutrality, by representatives of the companies it was supposed to regulate, a pattern of movement between industry and agency that one critical EPA scientist labeled the "revolving door."[26]

Yet even under such difficult circumstances, the EPA occasionally was able to enforce a regulation or fine a company. However, such successes actually added up to an unevenness of enforcement that exacerbated distributions of privilege and disadvantage.[27] The agency's tendency to levy its heaviest fines against those polluters near middle-class neighborhoods intensified widespread corporate strategies of instead locating garbage incinerators, dumps, and toxic-waste sites near working-class or underemployed neighborhoods, communities constituted through racialized and geographic arrangements of power.[28] In the early 1980s, African-American civil rights activists associated with the Washington-based United Church of Christ's Commission for Racial Justice gave this arrangement a name—"environmental racism." This term was defined as "racial prejudice plus power. Racism is the intentional or unintentional use of power to isolate, separate and exploit others. . . . Racism confers certain privileges on and defends the dominant group, which in turn sustains and perpetuates racism. . . . Racism is more than just personal attitude; it is the institutionalized form of that attitude."[29] Analysts saw the concentration of pollution and hazard in the neighborhoods of African Americans and other disenfranchised groups as a continuation of government-sanctioned unequal distribution of services such as housing, education, and health care.

Unionizing EPA scientists knew about disenfranchised communities' efforts to represent environmental problems through a civil rights discourse that emphasized the racialized and unequal distribution of hazards. The inaugural incident of environmental justice activism in Warren County, North Carolina, for example, even included a few EPA scientists as rally speakers. Moreover, during the 1980s community environmental activists had lobbied the EPA ceaselessly to incorporate into their mandate environmental justice analyses of the racial distribution of hazardous waste.[30] Environmental justice critics of the EPA used civil rights legislation against inequality. Thus they employed a different strategy from earlier toxic-waste activists who had used popular epidemiology to demonstrate chemical exposure and trigger a state-sponsored scientific investigation or pursue toxic torts. These two forms of activism depended on different stances toward the state. Critics of environmental racism portrayed the state as historically complicit in the production of racialized inequalities, while toxic-waste activists tended to see the state as failing to secure protections that had been expectations in the past. What the movements shared, however, was a distrust of the EPA.

Caught between the activists' criticism and an antiregulation administration, a small group of EPA scientists, many with "backgrounds in environmental, political and labor activism," took the unusual and impressive step of organizing a union of "toxicologists, chemists, biologists, attorneys and other environmental professionals" in the name of scientific ethics.[31]

Thwarted Science

Chartered in 1983, the National Federation of Federal Employees (NFFE), Local 2050 represented approximately twelve hundred EPA professionals.[32] The leadership was primarily composed of left-leaning, white male senior scientists, many of whom had been with the agency since its inception, were dedicated environmentalists, often held strong antiracist beliefs, and had risked their jobs as outspoken critics of EPA positions. The union argued that as government scientists they had "a duty and a right to perform our work in an ethical environment, and to see that our work is not distorted, misrepresented, stolen or lied about in devising false cover for Agency policies."[33] Their professional ethics, they argued, were being corrupted through the influence of "economically powerful industries that are doing things harmful to the environment."[34] They claimed a lost "right" to a neutral work environment. The union's criticism was very much like that of toxic-waste activists.

Through the union, EPA scientists fashioned themselves as champions of objectivity and as spokespersons for nature.[35] The particular version of objectivity they upheld was the common garden variety in modern Western science, what Donna Haraway has called the "view from nowhere," which relied on scientists to act as "modest witnesses" who kept the details of their persons separate from the practice of their science.[36] This particular construction of objectivity dovetailed with the way white privilege functioned in postwar America—both relied on holding an unmarked and neutral location. Though this type of objectivity had its historical roots in white privilege, its upholders were by no means necessarily racists. Though a "view from nowhere" was produced by and supported racialized privilege, it was not necessarily a conservative ideology. It could also be deployed in a liberal frame to argue for the desegregation of science by asserting that the race, sex, class, or religion of a scientist was irrelevant to the scientific method. In positioning themselves as defenders of objective science, members of Local 2050 complained not of a disruption of the neutrality of their identities but rather of a violation by the EPA administration to the neutrality of their workplace. As civil servants working for the nation's citizens, they had a "right" to a disinterested workplace in which they could execute their duty.

The union blamed the corruption of science in the EPA on the influence of large companies and industry-sponsored organizations over everything from the agency's promotions, to its research agendas, to the wording of its reports and brochures. The presence of corporate interests in environmental science even extended to experimental design and practice at the EPA. As practitioners of toxicological studies, the scientists knew that tinkering with humidity levels, changing strains of mice, modifying forms, or using stationary, rather than body-mounted, air samplers could determine whether a chemical exposure was detected or remained invisible.[37] They also knew that corporate scientists were expert at these manipulations.

EPA administrators could be both flagrant and subtle in obstructing their own scientists. At their most flagrant, administrators would prevent scientists from going public with findings critical of large corporations. Anyone who went ahead risked ruining his or her career. At their subtlest, EPA administrators could counter almost any positive finding made by an EPA scientist by pointing to a nearly identical, corporate-sponsored experiment that produced a negative or more ambivalent result. Uncertainty justified yet more studies and the continuing tinkering with protocols. Ceaseless calls for more studies allowed the production of ever more ambiguities and thus the generation of uncertainty ad infinitum, helping to make regulation next to impossible.

This purposeful production of uncertainty was indeed the subtlest means of distorting the founding goals of the agency and serving the antiregulation agenda. The union fought to counter such tactics, as illustrated by its resistance to the production of uncertainty in its struggle with the EPA policy on the potential toxicity of new carpet.[38] The union went so far as to videotape an experiment at Anderson Laboratories, one of the few independent toxicology labs in the United States. By blowing air over the carpet and onto mice, Anderson found that some carpet samples caused severe neurological and neuromuscular reactions.[39] The EPA, charged by Congress to attempt to replicate the study, reported that it could not. Likewise the carpet and rug industry also reported a failure to replicate Anderson's findings. Both of these experiments subtly modified the apparatus. Instead of blowing atmospheric air, as the independent lab had, they used bottled air and then bubbled it through water before it blew onto the mice, arguing that this provided a more controlled and thus better protocol.[40] This experiment, despite its slight difference in setup, found the independent lab's findings unreplicatable.[41] In the end, the union could not successfully subvert the development of the EPA's industry-friendly "green tag" carpet program.

In the late twentieth century, the extreme difficulty of making visible the health consequences of chemicals became the single most significant characteristic of "chemical exposures" as a scientific artifact. Yet rather than locating the problem in the way the EPA attempted to resolve questions of chemical exposure—that is, on the narrow terrain of laboratory toxicology—union members largely sought to hold on to the terms of their scientific practice by critiquing the conditions under which it occurred.

The formation of Local 2050, however, was predominantly motivated by the scientists' defense of state scientific practice against corporate interests. Though exceptional in many ways, their workplace activism was also a part of a late-twentieth-century swell in unionization among government and office workers, one that went against the tide of a waning and beleaguered industrial labor movement. Through unionization, scientists were recognizing their devalued status. No longer glorified as the influential and disinterested arbiters of disputes between

citizens and corporations about the consequences of industrial pollution, EPA scientists implicitly aligned themselves with the downtrodden,
proletarianized service sector rather than with the upper administration's managerial class. Thus, the way they expressed their activism and
its protection of objectivity was partially predicated on the conflicted
assumption of a subjugated position in an era of undermined white
privilege. Yet their ideology was the inverse of epistemological claims
made in terms of identity politics (including feminist arguments), which
typically argued that subjugated viewpoints provided better access to the
truth.[42] Instead, the officers of Local 2050 saw their oppressive circumstances as disturbing the neutral ground they held as necessary for the
production of good science.

Environmental Anxiety

As a union concerned with workplace conditions, Local 2050 soon became focused on not just the political but also the environmental conditions in the agency's headquarters. The local turned its attention to
Waterside Mall just at the moment when there was a nationwide surge of
distress over the unexpected presence of chemical exposures inside office
buildings. EPA scientists, whose very livelihoods connected the politics of
environmental exposure and suspended perceptions, were not immune
to this distress or to the way privilege shaped its articulation.

Pervasive white privilege was imperfect and insecure in a cold war
period as much about emancipation and civil rights as about conservative
containment.[43] Whites were losing the geographic and workplace mo-
nopolies they had enjoyed before desegregation, while the intensification
of globalized capital flows in the 1980s saw U.S. industrial jobs moved
abroad and middle-class managerial jobs downsized. Anxiety triggered
by new forms of insecurity abounded (and were brilliantly satirized by
DeLillo), helping to create a middle-class "risk society" worried over
errant chemical exposures that violated expected protections.[44] Chemical
exposures were not confined to factories. They could come from consumer products, construction materials, passing luxury vehicles, perfect
green lawns, designer pharmaceuticals, shiny blemish-free apples, or
plush carpets. Objects that were the very hallmarks of suburban privilege
could let loose exposures that violated racialized protection.

The inability to absolutely contain chemical exposures through privilege prompted many middle-class Americans to ask nervously, "Is it happening here?" On the one hand, the regularity and expectedness of distributions of racialized privilege made it possible to displace unearned privilege onto the naturalness of place—bad things happen to people in low-lying areas or in scrubby parts of the country. Better yet, chemical accidents happened to people who lived in faraway places, such as Bhopal.[45] On the other hand, illnesses such as breast cancer and leukemia indicated that no one was absolutely safe. While the environmental justice movement highlighted raced and classed distributions of toxic exposure, white middle-class America expressed its own version of environmental politics by seeking to isolate and prohibit all dangers, no matter how small, from the home, road, playground, and workplace. Thus not only were exposures themselves racialized and classed, but so, too, were environmental anxieties, shaped by an insecure yet pervasive white privilege.

The EPA headquarters was ripe to be identified as a "sick building" and environmental hazard. Under Reagan, physical conditions at the Waterside Mall epitomized adverse workplace circumstances.[46] Approximately five thousand agency staff members now crowded inside. A jumble of hallways led to a crazy quilt of tiny individual offices, most without windows, cut out of what had originally been apartments, creating a "warren of people crammed into rooms." In typical energy-efficient construction, those windows that did exist were unopenable. The building's interior was filthy and neglected: roaches and mice infested the offices, burned-out light fixtures left corridors dark for days, and toilets were often out of order. The air was stale and vent grills were clogged with debris, grit, and fibrous matter that caused a fine black powder to settle on surfaces. In the words of its inhabitants, the building was "oppressive" and "a dull, dirty, and depressing place to work." One EPA manager compared it to conditions of disadvantage outside the headquarters' door, writing, "I understand how poor housing project occupants feel," while another employee dramatically likened the conditions to ones in "Third World public hospitals."[47]

The administration tried to give the building a quick facelift by installing new carpet in 1987. Immediately, some EPA staff, including scientists, began to complain of acute symptoms: tearing eyes, irritated throats, burning lungs, shortness of breath, crippling headaches, and dizziness.[48] As the carpet installation pushed its way through the building, the trickle of complaints turned into a torrent. The EPA's Emergency Response "SWAT" Team, usually held in reserve for toxic spills, was called in. The facilities management director reported the results at a staff meeting: though sixty-eight different airborne chemicals had been detected, all were at concentrations "no more higher [sic] than your living room."[49] EPA scientists found themselves facing the same regime of imperceptibility that their own fieldwork had participated in.

Local 2050 became consumed with the issue of "indoor air quality." Members channeled their challenge of corrupted science into proving the existence of harmful chemical exposures in their own workplace. Union leaders fashioned themselves as defenders of the victims of exposure among their own. With their expert technical skills, EPA scientists had a unique insider opportunity to demonstrate how the detection of harmful exposures was purposefully avoided or, in other words, how suspensions of perception had been strategically generated at the agency.

Some of the sickest and most outraged employees formed the Committee of Poisoned Employees (COPE). With NFFE Local 2050 and the American Federation of Government Employees (AFGE) Local 3331— which represented clerical and other workers in the headquarters, many of them women and persons of color—they organized a protest outside the building in May 1988. Approximately sixty employees assembled there, carrying signs festooned with upside-down EPA logos or declaring "EPA is a Superfund Site." Inspired by toxic-waste-activist practices of popular epidemiology, Local 2050 handed out a survey. Out of necessity, but not without a sense of drama, some of the sickest employees had begun wearing gas masks to work. Placards reading "Canaries in a Coal Mine" underlined the belief that if chemical exposures could be found in white-collar workplaces, they might occur anywhere. Office buildings were "ordinary" and unmarked places, that is, places where privilege was expected to operate and where systematic disadvantage was expected to be rare. Moreover, carpet was a ubiquitous artifact of contemporary living and might be found in almost any kind of building. A chemical exposure through carpet at the EPA headquarters, of all places, simultaneously signaled the subjugation of agency workers under Reagan and the lack of immunity that privilege was providing more generally. The irony of this expression of environmental anxiety quickly captured media and Congressional attention.

Local 2050's protest tactics stood in sharp contrast to official EPA policy on indoor exposures. The EPA had, under duress, recently established an Indoor Air Division, which remained silent about the events happening in its own building. In general, the Indoor Air Division used the term "indoor pollution" as a discursive strategy to remove the problem of chemical exposures in nonindustrial workplaces from the realm of labor disputes and possible regulation. The division had been added by Congress in response to a large-scale study of "total exposures," which measured accumulated personal chemical bombardments.[50] The study, headed by EPA scientist Lance Wallace, had unexpectedly concluded that time spent indoors, not proximity to industrial sites, was most strongly correlated with high accumulated exposures. While this study was silent about the social locations of its research subjects— university students—and thus the possible effects privilege might have on the significance of indoor exposures, it did move the white noise of errant chemicals in "ordinary" spaces into the realm of perception, if only momentarily. Because of this study, Wallace acquired a reputation as the "father" of indoor air pollution.

In response to Local 2050's lobbying, Wallace headed a study of Waterside Mall. Almost two years had passed since the carpet had first been laid and the building had been aired out many times since. Any acute emissions from the carpet were long gone. Provided only with funding for stationary air monitors, Wallace expected to detect little: "More monitoring wouldn't have told us anything anyway. We were there a year after the fact and even studies where people have gotten there fairly quickly tend to fail to show anything."[51] Months after the initial complaints, air sampling measured no acute doses of a specific chemical, and therefore no acute chemical signal could be found amid the daily noise.

Predicting that no physical evidence would be found, the study also included an elaborate questionnaire, which had been given to all EPA employees in the building and had elicited 3,955 responses. Trained in atmospheric physics, not sociology, Wallace (like the "housewives" turned toxic-waste activists who practiced popular epidemiology) found himself spending his days analyzing a survey, assembling hundreds of pages of quantitative analysis, eventually published in four volumes between 1989 and 1991.[52] Ultimately, however, the survey allowed Wallace only to remark on the high prevalence of health symptoms at the

EPA. No single cause could be extracted from the white noise of Waterside Mall. The search for a single cause generated imperceptibility in two mutually constitutive directions. First, any specific single exposure years ago was masked by the complex and accumulated bombardments, both social and physical, to which inhabitants of Waterside Mall were regularly subjected. Second, the environmental study designed as a search for a single toxic culprit obscured the social and political circumstances through which the EPA site had become so degraded.

Local 2050 doggedly persevered in its attempts to make visible the antagonistic workplace conditions under which the study was conducted. Invoking a clause in their collective bargaining agreement that guaranteed a role for EPA scientists/union members in studies of their own workplaces, they added a supplement to the published findings. Agency internal memos, newspaper articles, earlier monitoring attempts, and independent research on carpet filled the appendix. By publishing these documents, Local 2050 sought to reframe the study in terms of the political conditions of its production. The lack of conclusion about the toxicity of carpet, which otherwise would have scripted indoor chemical exposure into its typical role of imperception, instead was held up as an example of the effects of corruption on EPA science. For Local 2050, at least, the administration's maneuverings within the EPA were laid bare in the appendix.

Meanwhile, six of the sickest EPA employees sued the building's owner. At first, the jury awarded them $948,000 in damages, the biggest indoor pollution award at that time. As with many other claims of low-level indoor chemical exposures made by the relatively privileged and disadvantaged alike, the defense reframed the scientists' illnesses as the result of anxiety—a psychological rather than a physical response. In 1995, the District of Columbia Superior Court overturned the damages, ruling that the building's owner could not be held responsible for psychogenic illnesses.[53] Not even their professional authority as EPA scientists could effectively give witness to the ill-health effects of toxic exposures occurring in their own bodies. Their claims were struck down with the same dismissal of hysteria usually saved for women and soldiers. The ground of professional authority and privilege shifted beneath their feet.

The scientists-turned-activists of Local 2050 had fashioned themselves as objective producers of knowledge because they believed their laboratory and technical procedures could disassociate them from the power relations swirling through questions of chemical toxicity. Forming a union in defense of the scientific ethics in the face of Reaganomics, the actions of Local 2050 were an exceptional and even radical act for a group of scientists who saw themselves as defenders of objectivity. Their outspoken criticism of corporate influence on state science was exceptional in an era of intensified boosterism for economic over environmental calculations of benefit and risk. Union leaders and the whistleblowers they defended persistently criticized official EPA findings before numerous Congressional hearings on such issues as fluoride, asbestos, and aerosol propellants. Yet the members of Local 2050 did not publicly question the technical terms of their scientific practice, just its context. As a result, what became imperceptible were the ways chronic and low-level chemical exposures, as well as their uneven distribution, were consistently rendered invisible by the narrow criteria of toxicological proof that their discipline, their agency, and the courts had developed—even when scientists worked to the best of their abilities and in good faith.

Seeing Race at the EPA

While Jack Gladney, the privileged protagonist of *White Noise*, had a hard time envisioning himself fleeing from a toxic airborne event, other people had less trouble recognizing their vulnerability to toxic exposures. With the rise of the environmental justice movement, reports by government scientists were regularly pitted against claims made by laypeople whose views of the world were shaped by a structural analysis of their disenfranchised position.

Much changed at the EPA in the years following the formation of the union. During President Bill Clinton's administration, the number of "minorities" working in Grades 13 and higher at the agency nationally more than doubled from 1,086 in 1993 to 2,348 in 2000.[54] The EPA headquarters' staff moved out of Waterside Mall in 1998 and, ironically, into the new Ronald Reagan Building. The departure of almost five thousand EPA employees from Waterside Mall left it empty and in danger of dereliction. Local Congresswoman Eleanor Holmes Norton compared the economic impact of EPA's departure on the Southwest neigh-

borhood to that of a "military base closure."[55] After considerable effort
by environmental justice activists, Clinton signed an executive order in
1994 mandating that the agency develop "environmental justice strategies," including use of Title VI of the Civil Rights Act of 1964, which
prohibited federal agencies from discriminating on the basis of race,
color, or national origin. Before long, a group of African-American EPA
scientists and staff charged that endemic and virulent racism existed *in*
the agency's headquarters. Scientists were finally naming the work of
race that had been inside all along.

Marsha Coleman-Adebayo, an African-American senior policy analyst
at the agency and an expert in African studies, sued the EPA on grounds
of racial and gender discrimination, winning a $600,000 settlement.[56]
The Republican-chaired House Committee on Science was quick to hold
a hearing titled "Intolerance at EPA: Harming People, Harming Science?" At the hearing, the NAACP came forward with the disturbing case
of another EPA employee, a mid-level administrator and African-American woman, who had been ordered by her manager to clean a toilet in
preparation for a visit from Carol Browner, the EPA's head administrator
under Clinton.[57] In her testimony, Coleman-Adebayo compared the EPA
to a "21rst century plantation."[58]

Coleman-Adebayo and a handful of others established a new activist
organization for EPA employees, the EPA Victims against Racial Discrimination (EPAVRD). Describing itself as "walking the last mile to
freedom," EPAVRD voiced its activism through the discourse and strategies well known from the early phase of the civil rights movement and
its social gospel Christianity. The group even enrolled Rev. Al Sharpton
in its protests and referred to Coleman-Adebayo as the "Rosa Parks of
the EPA."[59] In contrast to Local 2050, EPAVRD strongly linked hostile
workplace conditions to long-standing prejudice against African Americans and women, not to the administration's deregulation ideology or
corporate influence. Moreover, the group charged that systemic racism
enacted by some of their peers not only discriminated against individuals but also distorted the agency's work. How could the EPA hope to
address environmental racism when the agency itself was racist? For
EPAVRD, discrimination against African-American scientists was a manifestation of the same discrimination that produced racialized distributions of hazard.

EPAVRD saw the government as complicit in the historically continuous performance of discrimination. Instead of playing out its opposition in the details of science as Local 2050 had, EPAVRD lobbied for a legislative change that would constrain the government itself. It dubbed the legislation "the first civil rights law of the 21rst century." The NO FEAR bill (Notification of Federal Employees Anti-discrimination and Retaliation Act) was a legislative strategy to protect minority government employees within government agencies from discrimination. Though the lobbying and press coverage in favor of this bill overwhelmingly focused on racial discrimination, tucked into the legislation was protection for whistle-blowers.

The NO FEAR bill enjoyed bipartisan support in a way no critique of corporate influence could. It was premised on deterring discrimination by making agencies pay the money for settlements out of their budgets, where as previously the money had come out of a common federal fund. In the preamble, preventing discrimination and protecting whistle-blowers was defended on the basis that "good science requires a tolerance of opposing viewpoints."[60] The implicit argument was that subjugated standpoints, from African-American scientists, for example, provided valuable "viewpoints" that differed from those produced when one insisted on a single "neutral" standpoint. Opposing "viewpoints" were necessary for the EPA to analyze environmental racism without prejudice. For EPAVRD, diverse subject positions were necessarily constitutive, rather than corrupting, of knowledge production. For EPAVRD, however, discrimination at the unsettled turn of the millennium was not an act reserved only for those who benefited from white privilege—senior black administrators were also the perpetrators of racism against their black colleagues. One's "race" and the way one exercised racialized arrangements were anything but a straightforward equation. The bill was signed into law by President George W. Bush on May 15, 2002.

In this chapter I have tried to show that racialized privilege shaped science in the 1980s, even when "race" was not explicit to the scientists' self-fashioning or their topics of study. The instability of white privilege and the authority of a "view from nowhere" in the late twentieth century were, I would argue, intimately connected during a historical moment when *what* one could see was increasingly linked to *where* one was seen to stand. The regimes of imperceptibility I have tried to link—the unmarked exercise of racialized privilege and the undetectability of chemical exposures in 1980s environmental science—did not just coexist, they en-

countered one another. The oppositional stances of Local 2050 and
EPAVRD enacted the work of race, one by drawing on the unspoken terms
of racialized privilege and the other by marking racialized disadvantage.
Local 2050 fought for the restoration of the right to a neutral workplace
without undue corporate or administration influence; EPAVRD fought for
civil rights protection against racial discrimination within the government, thereby fostering "opposing viewpoints."

Whether "race" was named or not, I have tried in this chapter to
understand it here, not as the property of individuals, but as a product of
uneven and changing distributions of privilege and disadvantage at the
end of the twentieth century. The work of race, seen and unseen, perme-
ated the day-to-day arrangements of science. It is important to underline
that the EPA was not exceptional or worse in this regard. In fact, if
anything can be said about the exceptional quality of EPA scientists, it is
how willing many of them were to become activists for scientific integ-
rity. I have discussed the work of racialized privilege at the agency as an
example of the pervasive force of race in all "normal" science. Race,
science, and chemical exposure were being made through each other
amid sedimented and yet shifting distributions of power that shaped not
just who was authorized to make knowledge, but also the very distributions of hazard being studied. These included the landscapes of chemical exposure that differed between a bourgeois mall and a maquiladora,
or between an office building and a hazardous waste dump. While
"race" may have been a subject rarely spoken about in the labs and
offices of the EPA in the 1980s, race wove the physical fabric of neighborhoods and office buildings, exposures and protections, questions and
methods that scientists lived with daily.

[6] **Crack open an office building** at the turn of the millennium and find a teeming ecology. Dust mites flourish in the carpet jungle, feeding on the skin flecks sloughed off by human workers. Nematodes and cockroaches inhabit its bowels. Buried in the walls, a cool spot condenses air moisture, forming first a drip, then a stagnant puddle populated by microbes and molds. Every morning a swarm of humans invades, introducing fresh batches of organisms and chemicals suspended in the "personal clouds" which surround their bodies.[1] The swarm is in constant motion, intense in the corridors but also maintained in a tide of small gestures in the hive of cubicles: a chair is nudged, fingers flail over a keyboard, a cup of coffee is raised. A piece of paper flutters to the floor, is caught up in a passing draft, swept into a vent, and sucked against a grate, creating a blockage. The chemical soup of molecules released from an ocean of office objects is disseminated by airflows, some held steady by mechanical ventilation, others transient, diverted by the angle of a partition or disrupted by a passing body. In some nooks and crannies the circulation finds a dead end, a reservoir in which the chemical soup gathers and intensifies. Crack open an office building and find an ecosystem that needs to be managed.

Office buildings in the late twentieth century were not just machines, workplaces, or sites of possible pollution, they were also ecologies—organic spaces that could become "sick buildings." Ventilation engineers, workers, industrial hygienists, and EPA scientists were joined by another newly minted professional—the private building investigator. Office buildings were not only the physical home of corporations, housing the practices that made up an important part of capitalism, they were also spaces that were themselves business opportunities. In the final two decades of the century, their maintenance became the province of for-profit specialized companies—building management and building inspection firms—that represented the interiors of buildings in ways amenable to visions of how capitalism itself operated. Moreover, the healthfulness of buildings was of deep interest to a selection of industries and their associations, most particularly the chemical, carpet, and tobacco industries. Ecology proved a very useful frame to this set of financially driven actors, each of which brought distinct motivations to the materialization of sick building syndrome. Ecology gave a framework for affirming the nonspecific and multiplous quality of sick building syndrome that was especially appealing to the tobacco industry, which actively resisted regulation. This chapter concludes that the concept of sick building syndrome achieved the prominence it did in the last two decades of the twentieth century largely because of the tobacco industry's efforts to promote an ecological and systems approach to indoor pollution.

Sick building syndrome would have looked very different without the cybernetically inflected ecology of the 1970s. *Ecology* was a word used to describe both a field of study (the scientific discipline of ecology) and an object of study (ecologies that existed in the world). Systems ecology took as its primary focus the study of the abstract patterns of relation between the organic and inorganic elements of a system. An emphasis on the management of the *system*, on the regulation of its flows, relationships, and second-order consequences, made systems ecology enormously attractive as a management ideology for business. This chapter traces how ecology was used to grant a complex, fluid, and multicausal form to business practices, building systems, and finally to sick building syndrome itself. The foregrounding of relationships defined by contingencies made ecological explanations extremely useful for assembling accounts that did not lay blame for indoor pollution on any one thing.

Systems Ecology

While the word *ecology* may evoke warm and fuzzy associations with environmentalism, green politics, and natural biotic communities, it is also a concept tightly joined to a capitalist imaginary, dating back to German zoologist Ernst Haeckel's nineteenth-century conception of an "economy of nature."[2] Ecology has always included within its purview both biological and nonbiological entities, and by the late twentieth century it drew on cybernetics to model the dynamic relationships among them. Systems ecology, in particular, was a branch of ecology that used general systems theory and cybernetics to map out the flows and cycles of ecosystems. Thus, it was a science that took as its primary focus patterns of relationships between elements and not the individual elements themselves. While biologists have long bickered over the true natural boundaries of ecologies, ecosystem ecologists of the late twentieth century, in contrast, held that "an ecosystem was not so much a concrete geographical entity as a flexible abstraction."[3]

The origins of systems ecology after the Second World War is closely associated with the inclusion of Yale ecologist G. Evelynn Hutchinson in the Macy Conferences on Cybernetics, in which participants from the biological, physical, social, and engineering sciences sought to enunciate a shared discourse on complex systems.[4] Hutchinson called for ecologists to study descriptively and mathematically how physical, chemical, geological, as well as organic entities formed self-regulating feedback cycles.[5] While Hutchinson considered ecologies to be complex, he also described them as bounded and stable communities. In contrast, Hutchinson's student, Howard Odum, together with his brother Eugene, developed the concept to describe open, changing systems composed of complexity that could not be explained by the sum of their parts. They claimed that levels of organization above the individual or the species could be discerned with the systems theory approach and the use of the circuit diagrams from electrical engineering to map "energy flows."[6] The circuit diagram represented the transfer of energy through processes that connected creatures, as well as the chemical, geochemical, and human features of an ecosystem. "In its structure and function," wrote Howard Odum, "nature consists of animals, plants, microorganisms, and human societies. These living parts are in turn joined by invisible pathways over which pass chemical materials that cycle around and around being used and reused and over which flow potential energies. . . . the network of these pathways forms an organized system from the parts."[7] The Odums populated ecosystems with pathways, flows, cycles, and networks, making up a "pattern of relations" that is the "structure of nature."[8] In his widely used textbook and elsewhere, Eugene Odum liked to cite the *Webster's Unabridged Dictionary's* definition of ecology: "the totality or pattern of relations between organisms and their environment."[9] Thus, ecosystems were not materialized as the collection of organisms and elements within them, but as the relationships and connections between populations and inorganic features.

The application of systems ecology spread beyond the study of natural communities. Systems ecology required "a hybrid with engineering, mathematics, operations research, cybernetics, and ecology" to take into its purview the "totality of man and environment."[10] Not only did humans play a role in ecosystems, but society itself could be understood as a complex cybernetic ecosystem, where cybernetics was understood as the "science of control."[11] Houses, industry, highways, agriculture, as well as the history of capitalism and religion could all be apprehended as ecosystems and represented through the circuit diagram (for a circuit diagram of the home as ecosystem, see Fig. 20).[12]

The management of ecosystems was made necessary by what Howard Odum called "the continual shakedown": "With the continual shakedown of order we cannot keep structures organized unless we continually restore order."[13] Odum's phrase described the tendency of systems to come apart or disorganize. If an ecosystem was not maintained, it would dissolve, and another system would eventually emerge. Moreover, once one understood how to manage ecosystems, they could also be engineered from scratch. Both Odums took this literally, working on the development of life support systems for humans: Howard experimented with artificial microcosms for NASA and Eugene wrote on space biology. With their emphasis on mapping and controlling relationships between the biological, social, and technological, the Odums declared ecosystems ecology a new managerial ethos for society.[14]

While it is more typical to link the history of ecology to the rise of late-twentieth-century environmentalism, management theorists also used ecosystem ecology to model corporations and markets. John Freeman and Michael Hannan founded the business field of "organizational ecology" in the late 1970s by transporting mathematical models of population ecology out of biology and into economics.[15] In organizational ecology, companies became organisms struggling to survive in larger ecologies, such as national markets, to which they had to adapt continually. In laissez-faire fashion, Hannan and Freeman believed that markets neither could nor should be controlled; instead corporations should gather information from which they could build diagrams, with which they, in turn, could develop strategies to adapt to "evolving" environments.

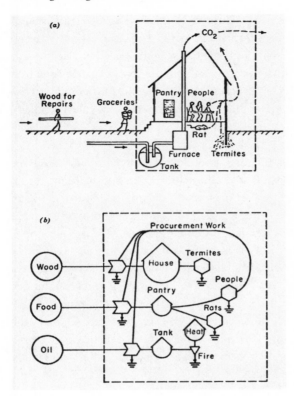

Figure 20.
Circuit diagram of human habitation involving energy sources, heating mechanics, human labor, and vermin. For Howard and Eugene Odum, systems ecology was a managerial ethos applicable to human society as much as nature. From Howard Odum, *Environment*.

By the 1990s, management books, seminars, and consulting firms regularly merged ecological metaphors with cybernetic principles to theorize how corporations could be "bioengineered" to "coevolve" in the "age of business ecosystems."[16] James Martin, for example, a business and technology consultant who was nominated for the Pulitzer Prize, extolled the concept of "cybercorp" (short for cybernetic corporation) as a combination of ecosystem and information technologies in his 1996 book, *Cybercorp: The New Business Revolution*. Martin's cybercorp was composed of an information technology "central nervous system" with "senses constantly alert, capable of reacting in real-time to changes in its environment."[17] A successful cybercorp was a "company resembling a living organism, all the parts are interconnected and interrelated. A healthy company is constantly growing and changing, adjusting to change in itself and its environment."[18] Martin's "cybercorp" vied for attention with a plethora of other management buzzwords all plugging into ecology and cybernetics. Similarly, in his *Managing the Information Ecology*, the information technology consultant and executive Bruce Hasenyager claimed that "information systems have become so complex and intertwined with process and politics that they now constitute an ecology."[19] Even Peter Drucker, perhaps the most influential American management theorist of the late twentieth century, called himself a "social ecologist."[20]

Office interiors, as important locations for business practice, were also increasingly apprehended as ecologies in need of management. Cybernetics-inspired studies of office communication patterns, for example, had led to the familiar "open-plan" office of the 1970s and 1980s. Circuit diagrams of communication flow continued to be used in the design of prestigious corporate headquarters, even if the typical open plan had degenerated into space-saving cubicle warrens. Another group of experts, human ecologists, also used the moniker "organizational ecology" to describe their approach to designing corporate interiors. According to Franklin Becker, a professor of human environment relations in Cornell's Department of Human Ecology, organizational ecology helped corporations "manage change" and "second-order consequences." Offices were "a system of loosely-coupled settings" and not "a box filled with different parts."[21]

Becker's version of organizational ecology drew from the work of Raymond Bauer, a psychologist and Harvard Business School professor who popularized cybernetics for business audiences with an emphasis on the management of "second-order consequences":

> The cybernetic model of system control is based on the assumption that one can achieve at best only some approximation of what he aims at. Therefore, salvation lies in rapid detection of error and adjustment to correct for that error.... this cybernetic model ... makes it natural to think of the second-order consequences of one's actions. "Error" is not a rare phenomenon that occurs because of bad planning and inept control. It is the natural and inevitable outcome of all purposive action.[22]

Control, in a cybernetic sense and contrary to the way it was emphasized in the interwar years, was not the precise generation of a static, standardized environment, but instead a set of managed responses to a dynamic and imperfect environment. Elaborating on Bauer, Becker held that office buildings took on a life of their own after installation, at a level of organization independent from specific participants and parts. This "life," made up of complex and changing relations, would inevitably result in unintentional events that were not errors but the nature of ecologies. It was just such second-order consequences, I will argue in this chapter, that became characteristic of a sick building.

Organizational ecology and similar office design systems were marketed as a means to control change, flexibility, and transience, often by abandoning the traditional practice of assigning each worker a single function and location. Instead, the "information worker" became a member of a transitory "team," which was formed, disbanded, and reconfigured into other teams. To organize work in this way, Becker promoted the briefly fashionable "nonterritorial office," in which flexibility was achieved, not by rearranging the furniture, but by rearranging workers in unassigned space. In the abundant business literature of the 1990s, nonterritorial offices and teams were described in futuristic terms: "The future will see more teams that function as amoebae—expanding and contracting, blurring both the center and the boundaries. Teams will be disposable, sometimes lasting only several hours; they'll be wholly elastic, coming in all sizes, and people will slip in and out of them instantly. And office designs will accommodate these ever changing teams: Flexibility, spontaneity, and the need to be fluid applies to the physical environment as well as to work processes."[23] Through organizational ecology, office buildings became sites characterized by fluidity, spontaneity, and process, qualities that needed to be manipulated and physically managed.

Applying ecology to the management of companies seems at times outlandish. Yet organization ecology was employed to design the offices of large companies such as Eastman Kodak, General Electric, Steelcase, Union Carbide, and Citibank. At its New York headquarters, Steelcase—an influential and longtime manufacturer of office furniture and early retailer of modular furniture systems for open-plan offices—represented its new version of "worklife" through the swarming patterns of an ant colony: "teeming with activity, the lobby exhibit features thousands of live ants at work and represents work at its most organic level."[24] Office buildings had become animated patterns of complex relationships. They had become sites whose nature was constantly in a state of becoming.

And it was this becoming, composed of relationships, processes, and second-order consequences, that needed to be managed to ensure that office buildings fulfilled their function: promoting productivity.

Organic Buildings

Apprehending buildings as ecologies drew on a long architectural traditional of analogy between building functions and bodily functions.[25] The mechanical parts of building-machines were analogized to the organs of the human-machine. While in the first half of the twentieth century this analogy turned bodies into machines, in the later half of the century it made buildings into pulsating organisms. A building was "a complex system of interconnected and interdependent parts. Like our bodies that get dirty and must be cleaned, that shed skin and replace body tissue, a building's surfaces get dirty and must be cleaned, and they wear out and must be renewed. A building's lungs, so to speak—the mechanical ventilation system of fans, duct work, heating and cooling equipment, thermostats, pumps, and all—must be energized, nourished, and maintained."[26] The building's viscera were set into animated physiological life with attendant mortalities and vulnerabilities.

New scales and modes of vitality populated organic buildings. Ventilation systems, as the circulatory systems, became sites of possible deadly microbial infection. In 1976, a widely publicized, mysterious infection in a Philadelphia hotel claimed the lives of twenty-nine participants at an American Legion convention. The Centers for Disease Control's epidemiological detectives solved the case through prototypical shoe-leather epidemiology—they identified a specific pathogen infecting the hotel's ventilation system, a bacteria that became known as *Legionella pneumophila*.[27] A handful of other nonfatal infections—humidifier fever, Pontiac fever, and q fever—spread through air conditioners and ventilation systems.[28] *Stachybotrys* and other toxic molds, potentially deadly to children, grew in drywall, ceiling tiles, or other moist areas.

As sick building syndrome episodes proliferated in the 1990s, investigations identified communities of creatures that made buildings their regular habitat: cockroaches, aquatic nematodes, dust mites, *Flavobacterium*, *Pseudomoas aeruginosa*, *Thermophilicactinomyces vulgaris*, *Cladosporium*, *Gliocladium*, *Rhodotorula*, and *Aspergillus fumigatus*, to name just a few. While it was not new for Americans to be obsessed with ridding their homes of "germs" or exterminating vermin, in office building investigations microbes and microscopic insects became expected life-forms. Although life among these cohabiting creatures was not necessarily noticeable or unhealthful, in abundance they could emit unpleasant odors, trigger asthma attacks, and even cause hypersensitivity pneumonitis.[29] The building, thus, had become more than a mechanical box; it was host to myriad flora and fauna, wanted and unwanted. A microscopic scale of life, rather than organization by organs, brought vitality to architecture.

Late-twentieth-century human bodies had also become populated with microscopic and molecular features.[30] Present everywhere yet without precise location, T cells and macrophages were understood to be constantly reacting to the intrusions of an outside environment, often portrayed in terms of threatening and foreign microscopic dangers, both biological and chemical, invading an interior world of eat or be eaten.[31] The life-and-death dramas within immune systems were monitored by laboratory T cell counts and immunological assays that had become crucial trackers of sickness and health. It is not surprising, then, that building anatomies had also come to possess immune systems. Air filtration systems and ozone generators—appended to HVAC equipment in response to indoor pollution—were often anatomized by manufacturers as immune systems killing off unwanted bacteria, mold, and fungi, as well as filtering out particles circulating in ductwork. "The Odatus Immune System," read the Web site of the manufacturer of an air purification system, "parallels that of the human. It also seeks out harmful microorganisms (contaminants) throughout the entire building and destroys them."[32] Buildings needed immune systems because they were, as building-organisms, susceptible to infection by microorganisms and infiltration by pollutants.

In the mundane world of ventilation engineering, a perception of buildings as natural systems that had to be managed had reanimated the modernist vision of rationally and perfectly controlled machines. While from the 1950s through the 1970s ventilation advertisements emphasized mechanical or automatic qualities by displaying pictures of gleaming steel parts, by the 1990s such advertisements were more likely to depict a river's churning whitewater or a snow-capped mountain (see Fig. 21). Yet nature in these ads needed to be monitored and managed,

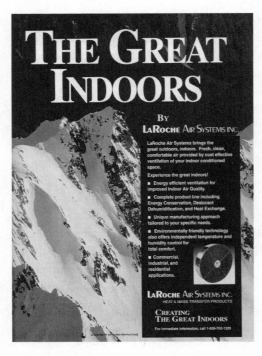

Figure 21. In the 1990s, ventilation equipment companies often portrayed buildings as natural spaces, in this case as "the great indoors." This was in contrast to the mid-century emphasis on buildings as machines that were automated and precisely controlled. *ASHRAE Journal*, December 1995.

not conserved and left pristine. The "great indoors" might be a natural system unamenable to perfect control, but it was nonetheless navigable with cybernetic building technologies.

By the last decade of the millennium, office buildings were not clockwork universes set in motion by rational engineering; instead their guts were complexes of organic and technological relationships that made up evolving ecologies. The building metamorphosed from a box that mechanically produced its "insides" into a cybernetic device that *managed* a teeming ecosystem within, sensing and adapting to the changing circulations and flows of technologies and organisms.

Buildings kept watchful eyes on the unpredictable ecology of the workplace equipped with a multitude of sensors: video cameras, thermostats, humidity sensors, motion detectors, light sensors, smoke detectors, and carbon monoxide alarms. Rather than a centralized "control console" in the basement operating at the "touch of a button," corporate buildings hired "facilities managers" who supervised a network of sensory feedback systems distributed throughout the building. Facilities managers did not operate a control panel themselves; instead, they managed a computer with specialized software that programmed the feed-back network of sensors and controls. Honeywell, a ventilation company founded in the nineteenth century whose other business interests included space, military, and industrial automation technologies, marketed its end-of-century equipment as an "open architecture" that can "give you boundless flexibility and freedom to expand and grow as needs change."[33] While the interwar building-machine had a closed mechanical structure composed of parts with specific functions interlocking in a static way, the end of the millennium open system managed change. In an open system, deviations from a "normal" environment were not perforce dysfunction; rather, they were the natural course of relationships and the inevitable consequence of adjustment.

As with air conditioning before the Second World War, only the most prestigious and newest buildings were installed as full-fledged cybernetic devices. More typical office buildings, though crammed with information technologies, still used the open-plan layout and modular air handling units established in the 1970s. Yet these buildings were still apprehendable as ecologies, as habitats to microbes, crisscrossed by chemical pathways, and staffed with "cyborg" workers hunched over keyboards and starring glassy-eyed at monitors, whose labor was extracted with little thought of their bodily "natures." When these workers began to protest the conditions in their office, savvy building managers called in not government investigators from NIOSH or the EPA but entrepreneurial building investigators, or "building ecologists."

Building Doctors and Building Ecologists

Using the tools of industrial hygiene, government occupational health investigators had been stumped by many sick building episodes. Only rarely could they prove that an episode had a specific physical, and not psychological, underpinning. Even if it was possible to find a contaminant in a particular building, government scientists were hemmed in by stormy federal regulatory politics: they were compelled to try to make specific causal connections and simultaneously limited in their ability to make those connections because their agency administrators wanted to avoid extending regulatory power into indoor spaces. Stuck between these constraints, government investigators rarely used the acausal and controversial explanation of sick building syndrome, leaving that term to private and university consultants.

Most building owners and employers eschewed government involvement in their properties and businesses. As facilities managers became more aware of how sick building episodes could disrupt production and provoke labor disputes, a market emerged for the services of private building investigators. In 1981, Hal Levin, a Santa Cruz, California, consultant, was the first American to mobilize the term *building ecology* to describe his services.[34] Ecology, Levin argued, allowed one to understand a building "as a dynamic and complex entity that continually changes in response to external conditions, occupant activities, and operation intervention."[35] A building's ecology, accordingly, was the result of the interconnectedness of people and things; a building exceeded its fixed structures and specific functions to include all the contingent interminglings inside it of people and paper, microorganisms and motions, chemical pathways and computer networks. Further, this ecology, despite the endurance of its glass and steel structures, consisted of an accumulation of transient and local relationships: the happenstance use of a highlighter pen or a colony of mold tucked under a carpet corner, for example. Because of these fluid and small-scale minglings, a single building also varied from moment to moment, and corner to corner. This accretion of continuously shifting relationships between organic and technological objects resulted in nonspecific building conditions that were both unpredictable and unamenable to techniques directed at predictable specificity.

These new private building investigators came from diverse backgrounds; they were engineers, physicists, chemists, university professors, and architects who used a pastiche of techniques to monitor both the mechanical and organic components of indoor environments. The appeal of the private building ecologists paralleled that of university industrial hygienists in the interwar years—they typically represented themselves as apolitical experts who could resolve labor disputes without government intervention. While building investigation firms were far from uniform, they shared a combination of entrepreneurship and ecological management that staked out a new subspecies of environmentalism specializing in indoor space. Concerned with apprehending the indoors as an *environment*, building investigators could sidestep simmering labor disputes: buildings were not dangerous workplaces in need of government regulation; they were ecologies that needed management techniques to keep them healthy.

Building ecologists, though almost never medical doctors themselves, often suggested a likeness between themselves and doctors. Building parts and diagnostic tools evoked the doctor-patient relationship in advertising imagery. In actual practice, building investigators drew on tools from clinical medicine to supplement the traditional instruments of industrial hygiene. Scopes at the end of long, flexible tubes gazed into ductwork or the space behind walls. Biological samples were taken from puddles; air conditioners and other moist places were tested at labs or with portable diagnostic kits. Building investigation companies had names like Pathway Diagnostics, Integrated Environmental Solutions, and Environmental Health and Engineering. In a sick building investigation, the building, not the workers within, was the patient in need of diagnosis.

One tool from the social sciences became commonplace in building investigations: the survey or questionnaire. The survey helped investigators make buildings their patients and workers indicators of a building's health. Surveys have already appeared several times in the course of this book, used as instruments for both consciousness raising and popular epidemiology. In both these uses, surveys assembled a *commonality* out of *experience* by making perceptible relations of proximity. When government industrial hygienists failed to find detectable causes or violations of ventilation codes to explain problem buildings, they, too, turned to questionnaires. Yet, for state scientists embroiled in regulatory politics, questionnaires were a second-rate tool, relying on data tinged with subjective assessments by disgruntled workers. As it became more and more customary for air samplers to come up empty-handed, the questionnaire, as the only piece of scientific apparatus providing positive results, came to be an end in itself. By the late 1980s, the questionnaire was established as the primary gauge for judging a building's health; it captured workers' symptoms, turning them into statistical data that, at least, could be fodder for analysis.

For private investigators, questionnaires were an important, but fraught, tool. On the one hand, building investigators, hired to quell labor unrest, worried over the ability of surveys to raise worker awareness: "Considerable caution must be exercised when interpreting subjective data such as the symptoms reported here. That is not to say that symptoms were imagined or contrived; however, when a population is made aware of a problem such as this, it is possible that this awareness increases the willingness of employees to report symptoms."[36] Realizing the power of questionnaires, many building managers were hesitant to let investigators use them, believing "it might alert non-affected employees, assuring liability or stimulating workman's compensation claims."[37] The Building Owners and Managers Association (BOMA), whose members manage the vast bulk of real estate with large offices in America, was particularly cautious about surveys. In Senate hearings on the Indoor Air Quality Act of 1988, both BOMA and the International Council of Shopping Centers testified against overinforming the public for fear of creating widespread panic.[38] Through careful design, however, subjectively reported data could be patrolled by the format of the questionnaire. Untranslated "experience" was threatening to both management and to the interpretive authority of the building investigator. Thus, very few questionnaires let the workers describe their "experience" in their own words; instead, the multiple-choice format was more typical.

On the other hand, questionnaires were attractive to investigators seeking to gauge the health of a building's ecology. Workers within buildings formed a readily available network of sensors, joining the thermostats and carbon monoxide monitors as registers of the state of a building. The prevalence and distribution of symptoms was increasingly held as one of the best indicators of a building's health, and questionnaires became the most telling instruments for reading worker-sensors. Workers were, "superior 'measures' to instruments, as they can provide an instantaneous summary of the long-term performance of the building environment whereas instruments can only measure the here and now."[39] The distribution of symptoms in a population provided the clues for how to adjust the building environment. Surveys, like ecosystems ecology, were able to materialize a troubled constellation of conditions in which buildings, not individual workers, were the survey's unit of analysis. Buildings as landscapes, not persons, were in need of care. Questionnaires could treat workers, not only as sensors, but as just one more contingency within the ecosystem.

Sick building syndrome itself became defined through the questionnaire. According to a widely used benchmark developed by the World Health Organization, a building was sick if over 20 percent of its occupants reported symptoms.[40] What made a building sick was the proportion of workers experiencing symptoms, not the kinds of symptoms or their cause.[41] "Syndrome" more generally denoted a concurrence of symptoms, not an event marked by a common disease or cause. A host of controversial illnesses at the end of the century were appended with the term: chronic fatigue syndrome, cumulative trauma syndrome, and Gulf War syndrome, just to name a few. The term *sick building syndrome* was sometimes accused of being a fraudulent or irrational term that hid the absence of a "thing" underneath it.[42] Such accusations expressed the discomfort of industrial hygienists and doctors who had identified symptoms as signs of some deeper regularity, such as a particular occupational disease or a particular chemical exposure. Sick building syndrome became a postmodern event "where there no longer exists any such 'deeper logic' for the surface to manifest and where the symptom has become its own disease."[43]

For private building investigators mobilizing the techniques of ecology, the imperceptibility of a single specific cause did not translate into the fraudulence of the event. As an ecology made up of a cumulative complex of causes, a building could lead to an array of unforeseeable effects and second-order consequences: the accumulation of low-level chemicals formed a noxious soup, which mixed with a long-gone transient airflow and contacted a stagnant reservoir, was compounded by a poor workstation and an oppressive managerial policy—there were so many contingencies that could go "wrong" in an office building. In short, "a complex of causes creates a condition that also has a complex of outcomes."[44] The power of ecology as a way of apprehending buildings was its ability to absorb contingency, accident, and uncertainty as its very nature. Workers symptoms and chemical concentrations were both rendered symptoms in a larger condition—the building.

Tobacco and the Building Systems Approach

Many private building investigators promoted their expertise in "healthy buildings," "building ecology," or "building wellness" as a means to manage buildings proactively through risk assessments, walkthrough inspections, preventive maintenance procedures, preplanning during building constructions, and regular "physicals."[45] Environmentally minded professionals designed "healthy buildings" or "green buildings" that used natural or other stable nonpolluting materials and were energy efficient. Other firms specialized in investigating and curing already existing problem buildings. However, more than just the expansion of environmentalism into the great indoors was at stake in their investigations. How firms identified the nature, and particularly the cause, of indoor pollution set the terms of its amelioration. If specific pollutants were the cause, they could be regulated. If workers' health was the object of concern, regulation might also be necessary. If a building ecology was the cause and the object of concern, its *correct management* was the cure, rather than the regulation of pollutants or the provision of health care for the individual.

In the 1980s, the largest building investigation company was Healthy Buildings International (HBI), located in Fairfax, Virginia. HBI had been a modest ventilation cleaning service called ACVA Atlantic until the Tobacco Institute, an industry lobby group, contacted its president, Gray Robertson.[46] Tobacco companies hoped to thwart the regulation of secondhand smoke in workplaces, restaurants, bars, and public spaces. Sick building syndrome appealed to the Tobacco Institute because it drew attention to the multiple causes of indoor pollution. Only a few cases of SBS had been attributed to tobacco smoke, a fact that Robertson, HBI, and the literature sponsored by the Tobacco Institute emphasized over and over.[47] Soon the Tobacco Institute and Philip Morris were building a database together on sick building syndrome cases, collecting a literature review, and contacting sympathetic indoor air quality experts who could spread news of sick building syndrome. In 1988, five big tobacco companies founded the nonprofit Center for Indoor Air Research (CIAR), which quickly became the largest nongovernmental source of funding for indoor air pollution studies.[48]

Robertson, with a monthly retainer from the Tobacco Institute, began to underbid other companies for lucrative building investigation contracts in the Washington area—the U.S. Capitol, the CIA headquarters, the Supreme Court, as well as corporate buildings on the East Coast such as the offices of IBM, MCI WorldCom, and Union Carbide.[49] Underwritten by Philip Morris, HBI expanded its scope by publishing a free glossy magazine that distributed over three hundred thousand copies in multiple languages.[50] The magazine promoted HBI's "building systems approach," which emphasized that "indoor pollutants themselves are not the root of the sick building problem. The real culprit often lies in the improper operation and maintenance and faulty design and construction of buildings, causing the structure to trap polluted air."[51] In short, indoor air quality problems were not about specific exposures and their health effects on individuals, but the "poor operation and maintenance of building systems."[52] In prose honed with the help of Tobacco Institute personnel, Robertson argued that "the accumulation of all pollutants are a symptom of these faults and not the cause of the problem."[53] While Robertson was promoting sick building syndrome on the road, his company continued collecting data that later became tobacco industry evidence demonstrating that secondhand smoke—unlike other culprits such as fungi, dust, humidity, bacteria, and formaldehyde—was rarely a problem in buildings.[54] His testimony before city councils, in court cases, and at federal hearings was pivotal to the tobacco industry's case that secondhand smoke was not a substantive indoor pollutant and thus not in need of regulation.[55] Framing indoor pollution in terms of buildings assessments rather than pollution also became standard at the EPA's Indoor Air Division, which labored under an antiregulation administration. Though scientists in the division successfully published a pamphlet declaring tobacco smoke a health hazard in 1989, one of the first official state declarations against secondhand smoke, the division in general strove for "consensus" with interested industries, foregrounding its own "building assessment" approach.[56] In practice, the management of building ecologies was collapsed into the management of building systems.

The building systems approach was articulated both to deflect attention from specific pollutants and to appeal to business and building managers. HBI promised to improve worker efficiency, reduce absenteeism, and save money without expensive redesign of buildings. Like many other firms serving the corporate market, HBI sold protection "from liability" and assurance of a "productive environment."[57] Publicizing attention to the environment "can be leveraged as a valuable communications and marketing tool," HBI advised potential clients.[58] For companies hiring private building investigators, it was useful to materialize an environmental problem, not a labor issue, and their services as a form of environmentalism. HBI promised not only to ameliorate a problem but also to polish a corporation's image.

The Tobacco Institute sent Robertson on a national media tour in 1986 specifically to promote the concept of sick building syndrome.[59]

With his grandfatherly good looks and charming British drawl, Robertson diligently sounded the alarm of SBS in local radio, newspaper, and television interviews, billing himself the "Buildings Doctor." The wide use of *sick building syndrome* as a term is largely due to his media junkets. This effort was so successful that the Tobacco Institute launched similar promotions of SBS in Canada, Hong Kong, and Venezuela.

Healthy Buildings International was not the only building investigation company wooed by the tobacco industry, nor was the Tobacco Institute the only industry association invested in derailing possible regulation of indoor pollution.[60] The Business Council on Indoor Air, founded in 1988, represented industry sponsors such as Dow Chemical and Owens-Corning at fifteen thousand dollars for board membership. It too promoted a "building systems approach."[61] In addition, the Tobacco Industry Labor/Management Committee developed a presentation on indoor pollution for unions, creating a coast-to-coast roadshow that ran from 1988 to 1990.[62] Conferences, professional associations, and particularly newsletters proliferated in which industry-sponsored experts rubbed elbows with independent building investigators.

The appeal of sick building syndrome was that pollution and its effects could be materialized in a way impossible to regulate—as an unpredictable multiplicity. "Virtually every indoor decoration, building material or piece of furniture sheds some type of gaseous or particulate pollutant," testified Robertson.[63] In its manual for building managers, the EPA warned that indoor pollution was "the product of multiple influences, and attempts to bring problems under control do not always produce the expected results."[64] Managing complex relationships among many "factors" and "symptoms" replaced a "naïve," "single-minded," and even "dangerous" attention to specific pollutants.[65]

The Dangers of Multiplicity

In a teeming building ecosystem, a discrete specific cause was extremely difficult and often impossible to track. A transient toxic plume could waft from an office photocopier through an air duct to the workstation of a distant worker, causing her body to launch an immunological response that she described as a headache. A moment later, however, the plume might move on or even disappear, called into and out of a fleeting existence by a set of events that may never repeat. Weeks later, an investigator with an air sampler would fail to detect any chemical cause and be left wondering if anything had happened at all.

The practical difficulty of tracing direct causal pathways from individual contaminants to individual workers opened the door to a philosophically sophisticated account of causal complexity. The sick building syndrome diagnosis and the building system approach highlighted the dangers produced by complexity: unpredictable health effects result when one combines numerous chemical compounds with crowds of microorganisms in busy spaces. In emphasizing matrixes of relationships, accounts of sick building syndrome drew on an ecological tradition in business and building management for support. Single, linear causal narratives were inadequate; change and adjustment were compulsory.

The terms by which sick building syndrome was granted existence, I have argued, were the result of a contested ontological politics. Women office workers, toxicologists, investigators, tobacco companies, and state scientists all advanced differing views on the nature of indoor exposures, populating them with divergent and even contradictory qualities. Surveys were the primary practice through which sick building syndrome symptoms were captured, and therefore surveys were important tools in the assemblages that materialized problems as multiplicities. For workers confronted with the limits of causal specificity, a survey could evoke a common event out of a community's differences. In this way, a survey materialized a community with multiple reactions to the synergistic effects of unequally distributed hazards. For building investigators, in contrast, a survey could demonstrate the impossibility of specificity within an untamable ecology. Through ecology, workers and exposures became symptoms connected by pathways in a mismanaged building.

Discerned as a condition in which simple causes were impossible, sick building syndrome was a terrain on which politically opposing versions of causal complexity played out. Workers materialized sick building syndrome as a way to hold employers accountable for the diverse corporeal effects of relatively privileged circumstances. But in the end, they lost control of the capacities of surveys and of the diagnosis itself. Thanks to industry advocacy groups, sick building syndrome became a means to disable accountability. Ecology helped to materialize other capacities opened up by multiplicity. Invoking multiplicity could shift the very grounds of causality to a constant uncertainty.

At a methodological level, as I have argued, sick building syndrome came to exist through multiple, sometimes conflicting, histories. This chapter has traced how multiplicity was itself one of the ways that historical actors brought sick buildings into being. That is, multiplicity was a quality with which objects, like buildings, could be imbued. The implication is that multiplicity was not a quality that could be simply celebrated for its eschewing of reductionism and embracing of diversity. Materializing an object as a multiplicity allowed historical actors to do concrete things about chemical exposures; at the same time, it disallowed and excluded other actions. It was precisely this capacity to exclude specific causal narratives and affirm ambiguity that made ecology and multiplicity such powerful ways to manage the physical corridors of capitalism.

[7] **You are inside** most of the time. Inside at work, at home, at the mall, even when you are on the move inside a car, bus, or plane. The inside, brought about by the built environments of late capitalism, provides your habitat, the milieu for your embodiment. Then one otherwise ordinary day your throat begins to constrict when you enter your newly renovated office building. Or your chest tightens at the photocopier. Or you notice that you have been overwhelmingly fatigued and foggy since they fumigated your apartment. A nebulous constellation of symptoms grips your body and will not let go. Your doctor cannot find anything wrong, yet your body seems to have run amok. The built environment that shelters your daily life becomes the site of your suffering. Bewilderingly, painfully, against all logic, your body seems to be rebelling against the inside.

The affliction of environmental illness, otherwise known as multiple chemical sensitivity (MCS), rendered the ordinary spaces of late capitalist life uninhabitable.[1] MCS brings together diverse individualized experiences of multiple symptoms that sufferers typically link to mild exposures of many unrelated chemicals. Like sick building syndrome, MCS is a phenomenon with a multiplicitous nature. Because individualized reactions are difficult, if not impossible, to objectify with conventional biomedical techniques and because they are elicited by low, subtoxic, supposedly safe levels of common, unrelated chemicals, the very existence of MCS was highly controversial in the late twentieth century, and it remains so. MCS does not conform to the biomedical logics already available for categorizing bodily states, nor does it conform to biomedical expectations of what a body is supposed to be able to do.

Conventional biomedicine greeted this newly emergent illness with more than skepticism—official associations of biomedicine have overwhelmingly proclaimed MCS to be an illegitimate diagnosis.[2] Facilitated by the predominance of women among MCS claimants, MCS was commonly rediagnosed as the *Diagnostic and Statistical Manual*'s somatoform disorder.[3] Many doctors saw promoters of MCS as charlatans taking advantage of the mentally ill. Through this diagnostic substitution MCS was categorized—usually against the patient's will—as a contemporary version of the age-old charge that women psychosomaticize their distress; in the 1990s symptoms took the form of chemical phobias instead of hysterical paralysis.[4] The irony in this diagnostic substitution was that somatoform disorders were themselves diagnosed as a collection of symptoms for which "no diagnosable general medical condition" could be found.[5] However, because somatoform disorders were understood as psychological rather than physical in cause, the lack of a specific causal mechanism did not render them illegitimate. Through this substitution MCS was removed from the realm of legitimate corporeal illnesses and became a gendered expression of psychological distress. The act of diagnosing psychosomatic illness instead of MCS was not just a simple renaming; it was a delegitimization that reverberated in workers' compensation systems, courtrooms, health insurance schedules, and other social institutions. MCS claimants had difficulty obtaining health insurance coverage, were ineligible for workers' benefits, could not gain workplace accommodation, found it virtually impossible to hold companies legally liable for their chemical exposure, and, perhaps most painfully, were suspected of malingering by acquaintances and even family.[6] The stigma around MCS was so great that sufferers could doubt their own claims of corporeal illness. The biomedical affirmation of the irreality of MCS multiplied into myriad juridical, state, and cultural domains, rendering MCS *abject*.

By abjection I mean the social, not psychological, process by which what was possible, intelligible, or material was designated by producing a domain of impossibility, nonsense, and immateriality. Abjection "designates 'unlivable' and 'uninhabitable' zones of social life which are nonetheless densely populated by those who are not enjoying the status of subject, but whose living under the sign of the 'unlivable' is required to circumscribe the domain of the subject."[7] Abjection was not simply a form of social exclusion. It made and marked a domain of supposed impossibility. MCS was abjected from biomedicine as a condition outside of "disease"—that is, as an invalid bodily state. Bodies with MCS were abjected not just from normality into abnormality but from the realm of possible corporeal abnormalities into impossibility. For that reason, one of MCS's most vociferous debunkers referred to it as a "nondisease," a term referring not to the presence of health, but to a nonmaterial form of suffering.[8] Sick bodies with MCS exceeded the possible, as designated by a conflux of mutually affirming dominant institutions for articulating illness, including biomedical diagnoses, courtroom precedents, and toxicology standards. Yet, if MCS could still be said to exist despite its abjection, then biomedicine's claim that it best understood the body could be undermined. Assertions of MCS as a simultaneously unintelligible and yet material experience threatened to expose the contingencies inherent in claims that a biomedical gaze adequately captured the body.

MCSers themselves commented on their abjection into densely populated "unlivable" zones in newsletters and support groups. They were " 'unbelongables,' those who are seen as uncomfortably different from some segment of society. Our illness/disability at times renders us, or makes us feel, Unbelongable in the mainstream society."[9] One MCSer called her illness "a beast," a second "a monster."[10] A third person wrote, "It is being treated like a 'thing' with 2 heads by the medical community —something that they can't explain and had rather not deal with because they cannot just write a prescription, collect their office visit fee, and be done with you; you are just a pain because you just WON'T get well."[11] They described themselves as "disposable cogs in a disposable world," "out of the equation," or as having "fallen through the cracks."[12] MCS was "like a one way ticket to the third world."[13] People with MCS lived with "rebellious bodies."[14] They were "the dispossessed."[15] As these descriptions show, the abjection of MCS was itself an additional horrible source of suffering.

The abjection of MCS was performed not only by biomedical and juridical institutions but also by some historical and cultural scholarship that was marshaled as evidence in courtroom testimonies and biomedical literature reviews that rejected MCS.[16] These debunking historical and cultural accounts have tended to presuppose that an illness's historicity is inversely proportional to its reality. That is, the more real an illness is, and the less culturally constructed, the more its qualities can be said to occur the same anytime, anywhere—the bacillus *Yersinia pestis* causes the plague regardless of historical setting and thus the plague is very real. In this way, "cultural construction" was used to explain only what biomedicine cannot. It presupposes that biomedical knowledge reflects the best truth of the body and is not itself also mired in historical sediments and limitations. Further, such works tended to accept uncritically the counterdiagnosis of psychosomaticism, relegating "cultural construction" to the realm of the psychological. History was thus confined to explaining only the form that psychosomaticism took in any given historical period—chemical phobias instead of paralysis, for example. Cultural constructivism was used in these instances to shore up abjection because it could perform a delegitimating or "dematerializing" effect. On the other side of the political spectrum, MCS advocates have often resisted abjection by uncritically accepting the terms that MCSers used when describing their illnesses as more authentic and truer accounts grounded in the unquestioned evidence of experience.[17] Calling for the recognition of MCS as a "real" illness has been the most tried and true route for advocates.[18]

This chapter is an experiment in forging another route through the quagmire around scholarship about abjected bodily states. I begin with the premise that both the terms by which MCS was abjected *and* the terms by which MCSers described their suffering were deeply historical. Even illness itself—what a body was supposed to be able to do, how it could be affected, how embodiment felt—was materialized in historically specific ways as an effect of power. How can a historical account affirm the materiality, or more accurately the materialization, of an already abjected condition? In this chapter I will endeavor to provide an account that interrogates, rather than supports, abjection.[19] As with sick building syndrome, I will set aside the question *Is it real?*—which has led too many accounts astray already—and instead start with the assumption that bodies are always multiply materialized in ways that do not exhaust the potential of future materializations. Further, though this chapter is itself an intervention in the debates surrounding MCS, I have focused my analysis on the material practices for managing bodies in space. How have bodies with MCS been materialized outside of their abjection from biomedicine?

An MCS Movement

A connection could begin at the health food store. Or you could meet someone in whom you recognized yourself. Then you bought a book, subscribed to a newsletter, or joined an Internet chat group. The everyday is heavy with the potential for new combinations. An abundance of lines ran through you, and, in the cultural fabric of late capitalism, there were myriad lives to be sewn. It was easy to find oneself dabbling in the alternative health movement. Despite the wall presented by managed care, alternative healthcare was quite common, especially for chronic illness. Americans spent about as much out-of-pocket money on it as they spent on conventional medical care.[20]

Alternative healthcare was itself fragmented into many different disciplines. What makes the term appropriate was not a shared set of practices or practitioners but rather a common outsider status. Each tradition of alternative health care could be called its own discipline or movement. Sick bodies enigmatically reacting to the built environment aggregated into what I will call the MCS movement.

This movement was not primarily a political one dedicated to protests and political actions, though certain cells within it were political in this way. It had neither an overarching goal nor a single charismatic leader. Even to speak of an "it" is a misnomer, for it lacked coherence. The movement was ad hoc, filled with people coping with illness at the level of the everyday, not with visionaries who knew their destination.[21] The movement was composed of participants who recognized something of themselves in each other. At the same time the movement cut across class and other social markers. Participants might never have met each other; they were geographically scattered and many only partially participated. One did not need to be a woman or even have MCS to join, yet the movement was primarily composed of women with MCS. Participants involved themselves to fluctuating degrees.

The MCS movement was formed of a network of informal cells where participants could come together: a newsletter, an Internet chat, a health-food store, a support group in a women's center, an understanding church, a specialist lawyer, an environmental illness clinic, a commune. I use the metaphor of cells to describe the movement because it was made up of many diverse pockets of activity that formed a supple tissue of contacts.[22] The movement held together a host of names and explanations given to sick bodies: environmental illness, chemical injury, immune dysregulation, twentieth-century disease, universal reactors, and multiple chemical sensitivity. Multiple chemical sensitivity was only the most repeated of these, though environmental illness was a close second. Besides the variety of names, there were many hypotheses to explain MCS, but most agreed that it was amorphous in its expression and nonspecific in its cause. Perhaps because multiplicity was signified in its name—MCS held together people who were injured by different chemicals and who reacted to many chemicals—it held together a multiplicity of symptoms and a multiplicity of causes. Symptoms were not only multitudinous but also varied from person to person. One might have suffered from brain fog, shortness of breath, fainting, dizziness, nausea, rashes, fatigue, moodiness, depression, loss of memory, slowed reflexes, or other conditions. Incitants might be any object found in late capitalist life. In its very manifestation, the illness was loose, explicitly envisioned as a field of variety.

This multiplicity extended to the movement itself; there was no single strategy, explanation, or instantiation. Some cells were oriented toward the political action of letter-writing campaigns, efforts to expose the industry backing of expert witnesses, or pursuits of government recognition. Some cells pulled on "new age" lines; others were fiercely Christian; some were organized around housing; others were an aggregation of trailers on an empty patch of desert land; some joined together in a lawsuit; others might be tested at the same laboratory; some worked together; others chatted in cyberspace.

At the end of the twentieth century, there were many such "new social movements," with a strength and robustness that came exactly from the suppleness of a cellular organization. New social movements in America around AIDS and Gulf War syndrome are good examples. Though they may have had in common certain qualities, or rather a certain lack of qualities, these movements were far from identical. The branch of AIDS activism represented by ACT UP, for example, was composed mostly of middle-class gay men who had access to financial resources and drew on a tradition of political activism from the gay and lesbian rights movement.[23] Because of the particularities of the illness, many of the participants experienced years of relative health, even if they were HIV positive. Unlike MCS, AIDS was an illness already being researched by biomedicine, and thus the movement was often aimed at critiquing and redirecting this research. The movement around Gulf War syndrome was also primarily composed of men, in this case soldiers and veterans.[24] Yet, like MCS, Gulf War syndrome was not embraced by biomedicine. Unlike the MCS movement, it mobilized an already existent infrastructure of veterans groups and had an obvious target for its political actions, the Department of Defense.

The MCS movement differed from these two movements in three fundamental ways. First, most MCSers were women, many of whom had difficulty maintaining steady employment once they became sick. Though MCSers often shared a common gender, the MCS movement lacked a coherent identity politics. The identity of "women," unlike that of "gay man" or "soldier," was rarely called on to hold cells together. Second, while some pockets of workers with MCS did have an obvious workplace target for their protests, the MCS movement in general had no obvious target; the kinds of chemical exposures MCSers recounted were not centralized around a single product or single polluter but were ubiquitous and ordinary. Finally, without a clear political foe, the strategies within the MCS movement tended to take on a different tenor, characterized by creating regimes for coping with unruly bodies in the everyday. It was through this experimentation with their own bodies and the spaces they inhabited that people with MCS built what I will call an "elsewhere within here."

Technologies of the Self and Elsewheres within Here

Imagine an "elsewhere within here" as a domain of presence that exists despite abjection. When we attend to the dense presence of people with MCS, it becomes clear that abjection was not absolute.[25] By taking notice of "elsewheres within here"—zones of "other" intelligibilities—the edifice of a single hegemonic biomedicine that alone renders what was possible and intelligible crumbles. Though marked as impossibilities, bodies with MCS were not abjected into an abyss of nothingness. Instead, bodies with MCS were captured by other connections and practices, producing new knots of possibility for inhabiting bodies, creating a densely populated elsewhere within here.

Abjection forced a *rematerialization*—of self, body, and illness—by people whose unruly bodies continued to react to the built environment. Rematerialization, however, was not just a simple matter of an incomplete expulsion, a leftover after the dominant ways of making sense of the world have cut you up and spit you out. Elsewheres within here were not just remainders; they were made at the often unexpected junctures

of other ways of apprehending bodies and environments. Just as an
elsewhere was densely inhabited, it was also intensely spun; one inter-
vened in the elsewhere even as one inhabited it.[26]

The MCS movement was composed of just such an accretion of small
actions performed in everyday life by people claiming to suffer from
MCS. I am not suggesting that these everyday practices were more authentic or accurate than the many scientific disciplines that this book has
already described; rather these practices were just as historically contingent. Nor was the everyday less complicated; it was messy, constituted
amid many possible ways for cutting up experience into categories and
multiple histories passing through bodies. At the same time, the "everyday" was typically composed of ordinary material culture and practices
around food, home, and body care that provided the texture for being a
person in late-twentieth-century America. The everyday was the site of
personal becomings where small modifications and detours sketched
out subject positions. Within the confusion of daily life people were
forced to cope with illness. The elsewhere of the MCS movement was
produced, not by great events, political maneuvering, or professional
articulations, but at the capillary level of inhabiting a sick body in a
particular historical circumstance.

This everyday agency tended to take the form of what Michel Foucault
called technologies of the self—caring, cultivating, sometimes destroy-
ing, always historically contingent and not universal—that permitted
people to effect by their own means, or with the help of others, a certain
number of operations on their own bodies, thoughts, conducts, and
ways of being.[27] The question *What can I do?* drove technologies of the
self. Pulling on practices already available, picking up tools, absorbing
objects, naming with new words, the self could be transformed and an
elsewhere constituted.[28] In the case of MCS, in occupying the position of
the impossibly disabled person and then naming this position as such,
there opened a possibility of subverting one's own invisibility.[29] In the
day-to-day inhabiting of an elsewhere, not only was the body rematerialized, but the incompleteness of abjection could be exposed. Exposing
how one inhabits a possibility designated as impossible could then be a
means of making other assemblages or climbing back onto old ones.

In the case of MCS, bodies reacting to the environment rendered it
pathogenic and the environment impacting bodies rendered them ill.

This juncture of mutual constitution provided grist for reconfiguring technologies of the self within the MCS movement. Further, there was a distinct gendering of this body/building nexus. First, the built environment guided and provided the milieu of acceptable gendered practices: the kitchen, the office, and the house as sites of women's work, or the pink room as the ladies room, for some obvious examples. Laundry detergents, bleaches, scrubs, and sanitizing aerosols were not only the equipment employed in caring for the domestic built environment; they also produced a gendered relation to that environment and a gendering of chemical exposure.[30] Second, this gendered caring extended to the body. In the drugstore one was confronted with cosmetics, diet supplements, magazines, "family" medicines, and other gendered tools for the micromanagement of bodies in end-of-the-millennium America.

People reacting to the cleaning chemicals, cosmetics, and building materials of domestic spaces did not simply reject this gendered body/building nexus, they called on it as the grist for their reconfiguration of an elsewhere. The actions of already gendered bodies drew on practices and objects, also already gendered, to trace out safe spaces and zones of habitability. Thus gender was not just coded onto people with MCS, they performed it. Turning from the question *Why is it women who mostly suffer from MCS?*, I want to ask, How did the gendered mutual embrace between bodies and the built environment become the site for building yourself a body in a safe space?

To sketch out how MCS was materialized in an "elsewhere," the rest of this chapter will empirically unpack strategies and practices that characterized many of the cells making up the MCS movement. My starting point will be the alternative practice of clinical ecology, a fringe medical field that has helped to articulate the concept of "biochemical individuality" on which MCS depends. I will then examine how biochemical individuality was manifested in everyday coping practices that sought to build "safe spaces." Safe space will then be followed into cyberspace, where an ethic of information exchange became a central strategy for linking up cells and individuals dispersed in space and isolated by their illness. Lastly, safe space will be linked to the body through the practice of micromanaging "body-ecologies," which were in turn largely populated by technoscientific objects. These various ingredients became the basis for experimenting with building yourself a body in a safe space.

Clinical Ecology

From its beginnings in the 1940s, clinical ecology was entangled with mental illness.[31] In a Chicago hospital, Theron Randolph, an allergist who specialized in food allergies and was soon to become the founder of clinical ecology, encountered female patients with mental illness who he believed were really suffering from food allergies. In a moment reminiscent of Jean Martin Charcot's presentations of hysterical performances at the Salpêtrière Hospital in Paris, Randolph filmed a severe four-day psychotic reaction induced by feeding his patient a food she was sensitive to—beet juice. The film lost him his position at the hospital, yet he continued this practice believing that many nebulous illnesses could be explained as sensitizations to common substances.

By 1965, Randolph and a handful of others founded the Society of Clinical Ecology, which defined its interests as the interaction between an individual and his or her immediate habitat as reflected in total health.[32] The environment that impinged on the body was distinctly the ordinary built environment of late capitalism. The goods, building materials, and pollutants of the late twentieth century joined its mass-produced foods at the top of the clinical ecologist's list of possible excitants in the personal ecologies of home and work.

With its ecological emphasis, clinical ecology deviated from two of the most influential scientific fields that studied the body's reaction to chemicals: allergy and toxicology. First, the field of allergy had become increasingly based on the identification of an immunologic mechanism centered on the artifact of immunoglobulin E (IgE), while its clinical practice was bound to mass-produced pharmaceuticals. Second, the field of toxicology had put in place its axiom of the dose response, in which every chemical had a characteristic and predictable effect on the human body only occurring at a certain dosage, the dose above which a chemical becomes toxic. The dose-response axiom held that the effects of chemical exposure were *specific* to the nature and amount of that chemical and *general* to all human bodies.

For clinical ecologists, allergy and toxicology were both examples of a problematic reductionism that compared unfavorably to their own ecological thinking. In forming their ecological vision, they drew on the systems ecology of Eugene Odum, who wrote, "A human being, for example, is not only a hierarchical system composed of organs, cells, enzymes systems, and genes as subsystems, but is also a component of supraindividual hierarchical systems such as populations, cultural systems, and ecosystems. . . . An important consequence of hierarchical organization is that as components or subsets are combined to produce larger functional wholes, new properties emerge that were not present or not evident at the next level below."[33] For Randolph, health was such an emergent property, a condition that constantly emerged in context and thus had to be investigated at the level of the ongoing interaction between body and environment.

Within this apprehension of health as an emergent property lay an articulation of an *individualized body* with a *personalized ecology*. In contrast to toxicological tenets, reactions were not specific to the chemical and general to the human body, but rather nonspecific to the chemical and individual to the body. No underlying mechanism or standard diagnostic test was necessary, or even possible, for clinical ecology practice. However, like toxicologists and ventilation engineers, clinical ecologists used the environmental chamber, but in a radically different way. They placed the patient in this chamber—understood as a chemical tabula rasa—into which they introduced low-level exposures.[34] The patient then subjectively reported any symptoms, mental or physical, provoked by each exposure. Acute reactions signaled a personal sensitivity to be avoided. Environmental chambers allowed clinical ecologists to isolate individualized, subjectively reported reactions to low levels of chemicals —a kind of reaction that lay outside toxicology's regime of perceptibility.

For toxicologists, the chemical effects that clinical ecologists postulated were nonsensical, and they were willing to testify as much in court. For allergists, if there was no IgE present in patient's blood, no allergic reaction could be objectified and nothing could be said to be taking place. Over the course of the 1980s, clinical ecologists became increasingly estranged from conventional medicine: medical organizations rejected them, insurance companies refused to pay their patients' bills, and judges no longer accepted their expert testimony in court. Perhaps because there was an increasing popular interest in clinical ecology and its practitioners were being called to testify in court cases regarding chemical exposure (and despite the fact that many clinical ecologists were also physicians) national medical associations came out with position papers in the mid-1980s critiquing its scientific merit. Strongest were the critiques by a select group of allergists and toxicologists with industry ties, the most outspoken of whom were Ronald Gots and Abba Terr. Both worked as expert witnesses against multiple chemical sensitivity claims and often appeared at conferences organized by the Environmental Sensitivities Research Institute, an industry-sponsored anti-MCS lobby organization.[35] Gots also founded the National Medical Advisory Service in Rockville, Maryland, which specialized in supplying expert testimony on behalf of insurance companies and manufacturers who confronted litigation about MCS, sick building syndrome, and other chemical injuries.[36] In fact, the now famous redefinition of the status of scientific evidence in the judicial system in *Daubert v. Merrill* was explicitly about clinical ecology.[37] While clinical ecologists began by claiming that mental illness was sometimes caused by food sensitivities, they ended up defending their diagnosis of chemical sensitivity against claims that it was only a cover for mental illness, that practitioners were tricking impressionable, mentally ill women into thinking they were chemically sensitive.

Fleeing an increasingly bad reputation, the Society for Clinical Ecology changed its name to the American Academy of Environmental Medicine. With clinical ecology's name change and the deaths of most of its founding members, the capital migrated from Chicago to William Rea's Environmental Health Center in Dallas.[38] The Environmental Health Center, a mecca for patients suffering from multiple chemical sensitivity in the 1990s, claimed to have treated over thirty thousand patients. The entire center was a gigantic environmental chamber of sorts. The walls were made of baked porcelain over steel, the furniture of hardwood or steel, the air filtered, the floors made of tiles, and computers and other equipment were enclosed in stainless steel boxes with separate ventilation. The center even rented "safe" condominiums for its out-of-town visitors.

While earlier clinical ecologists spurned conventional allergists' slavish reliance on an immunological mechanism, later clinical ecologists practiced their own form of "clinical immunology" in an attempt to objectify environmental illness and win scientific legitimacy. Using their own laboratory testing facilities, environmental medicine centers offered their patients a staggering array of immunological and brain-scan tests: antibody assay testing, activated lymphocyte profiles, autoimmune disease profiles, porphyrim enzymes, and single photon emission computed tomography (SPECT) scans, to name just a few. The body materialized at the molecular level became central to the reformulated practice of environmental medicine and a reformulated notion of bodily individuality, called biochemical individuality.

> Biochemical individuality of response is the individual's uniqueness. This uniqueness of response depends on the differing quantities of carbohydrates, fats, proteins, enzymes, vitamins, minerals, immune and enzyme detoxification parameters with which an individual is equipped to handle pollutant insults. These variations determine an individual's ability to process the noxious substances he encounters. . . . Thus, a group of individuals may be exposed to the same pollutant. One person may develop arthritis, one sinusitis, one diarrhea, one cystitis, one asthma, and one may remain apparently unaffected.[39]

By objectifying individuality with the biomedical techniques for assessing the molecular body, practitioners of environmental medicine hoped not only to help their patients but also to gain scientific acceptance. Still, their treatments remained nonpharmaceutical, instead drawing on a bricolage of alternative health approaches, from old-fashioned avoidance to programs of "detoxification." And like earlier clinical ecology, most of environmental medicine's patients were women.

Doctors, expensive lab tests, professional squabbles: by climbing into the history of clinical ecology, my narrative has strayed far from the everyday. Or has it? This detour has been necessary because "biochemical individuality" and "personal ecologies" became the objects that many people with MCS sought to care for. And in a way, many MCSers shared clinical ecology's desire for biomedical acceptance. Climb out of this cell and back into the confusing everyday of bodies struggling with the built environment. Clinical ecology was only one cell among many that MCSers connected themselves with to cope with their condition.

Space and Salvation

While clinical ecology was very concerned with its status in biomedicine, in the everyday MCSers were obsessed with the search for "safe" spaces within which their bodies would not react. If the chemically reactive person was to live with others, she or he must get them to modify spaces and change behaviors that were coded as benign by everyone else.[40] While some MCSers struggled for accommodation in their workplace, invoking the Americans with Disabilities Act, and others wore masks to protect themselves when they ventured out into the world, the search for safe space usually involved a retreat into the home.[41]

Safe space was personal; since all people possessed their own "individualized biochemistry," the exact contours of the safe environment were individually specific. Further, every space was already idiosyncratic, with its own constellation of objects creating its own atmospheric soup. Thus, the search for a safe space required the development of an individualized regime of self- and space care.

Domestic space, unlike workspace, was already personal.[42] In their quest for safe space, MCSers made the home into an individualized environmental chamber. Since the home and its tending were already gendered, it was this gendering that many people with MCS often called on in their search for salvation. The already gendered work of house care—mopping, disinfecting, scrubbing, dusting, tidying—was at the same time marshaled and reconfigured. Cleaning products produced exactly the kinds of common, low-level chemical exposures that MCSers reacted to, yet this corporeal rejection of the products did not translate into a rejection of the practices themselves. Housework—which may have been harnessed previously, and even obsessively, to the goals of ridding the environment of germs, making the floors sparkle, and doing laundry that glows whiter-than-white—was channeled into making the home chemical- and exposure-free.[43]

The ecosystem of the ordinary home was composed of its building materials, the products inside it, the microorganisms that lived in it, and the people who inhabited it. As with the labor of maintaining a spotless house, rehabilitating the corrupted home was labor-intensive and required establishing a great deal of control over the space. In this endeavor, the usual products for house cleaning and personal grooming became suspect as sources of possible chemical exposure. Even the materials that composed the furniture, walls, and floors—chipboards, vinyl, polyester, plastics—could be unsafe. A simple act such as buying the right shampoo became a serious undertaking. The ideal safe home was one in which the objects that composed it were not volatile—did not "off-gas" chemicals into the air—and thus did not strongly impinge on the body. To create such a space, walls were covered with steel foil, furniture was made of either steel or hardwood, and cotton replaced synthetic fabrics. Vinegar and baking soda substituted for chemical cleaners. Products with fragrance or people wearing perfume were banned. Since the home as ecosystem was constantly changing every time a new product was brought in, a guest arrived, or a window was opened, it had to be vigilantly managed.

The home rendered as ecosystem was not a gesture returning space back to a pristine nature, nor was it a Luddite or anticapitalist gesture. The built environment had to be remade as an "environmental" background. Yet, as with the management of an office building or a city park, marking off certain spaces as ecologies required management and work. All sorts of technologies were used: charcoal masks, air filters, water filters, ion generators, electromagnetic meters, and pollution detection kits were crucial tools for home management. While chemical cleaning products were rejected, other technologies replaced them. The gizmos and doodads for producing a safe space were traded in a market niche catering to this ecological management, a market which, moreover, was not confined to alienated MCSers but also included environmentally concerned middle-class consumers. One could proudly mark oneself as part of the MCS movement by purchasing hats, shirts, pins, and cards sporting pictures of the earth or a canary wearing a mask.[44] "Natural" or "safe" was a quality that could be listed on a product's label.

Creating and managing the "nature" of space was a time-consuming and difficult task. One could find many books and guides to help.[45] If you had the financial means, there were consultants who would do it for you: Tender Loving Care Environmental Consultants helped you over the phone, the Environmental Health Center of Dallas offered this service to individuals as a sideline, and professional building investigators did the same for corporate space. Most women, however, did it themselves. Even when the labor was your own, it was expensive to make a safe space and the sick person of meager means could easily fail. With their rebellious bodies and expulsion from health insurance coverage, many MCSers moved a rung down the economic ladder, sometimes becoming chronically unemployed and stranded in poverty.[46]

MCSers easily found themselves sleeping outside, living on the porch, or in the backyard. Unemployed, stigmatized as malingerers, suffering from mental and physical symptoms, unable to find an urban apartment with "safe" building materials, MCSers sometimes lived in their cars. The back pages of MCS newsletters were often reserved for people's pleas for safe space: "DISCOURAGED (2 YEARS IN A CAR)—EI [Envi-

ronmentally ill] needs living space—trailer space or cabin";[47] "Chemically sensitive women seeks others who can buy 1/3 or 1/4 share in an
EI-safe house. Willing to relocate";[48] "HOUSING NEEDED. 47 year old
woman with MCS wants to rent safe housing in the Portage or Madison,
WI areas."[49] The search for space often led people with MCS to abandon
urban spaces in favor of trailers parked in less polluted rural areas. Dry
places such as New Mexico, West Texas, Colorado, and Arizona were
particularly popular. Trailers in tow, they joined up to form small MCS
communities or chip in together to buy and make a safe commune. In
San Rafael, California, the Environmental Health Network founded a
HUD-sponsored housing project called "Ecology House." Cells sometimes organized around plans for possible MCS communities (Randolph
called them "ecolonies") in Kentucky, California, Oregan, Utah, Texas,
or Arizona.[50]

While biomedical critics commonly affiliate MCS with new-age spir-
itualism, there were actually more Christian cells, which explicitly invoked the Christian tradition of personal salvation. The "Alpha Omega
Christian Communities for the Chemically Ill" was a ministry in San
Antonio, Texas, that met in an outdoor chapel and was founded by a
woman for the chemically injured. Searching for both spiritual and
environmental salvation, the ministry drew on the American tradition of
linking salvation to new lands. Guided by the "Word from God," members sought to form a Christian community for the chemically injured,
called Eagle Ranch: "The Eagle Ranch is owned by no man, but by
Yahweh the God of the Bible. It exists because the Father ordained it,
Jesus came to live here and the Holy Spirit led people to donate time,
land, or money so His children, the chemically injured, may have a safe
place to live."[51] Safe space saves, both in the physical and spiritual realm.

The search for safe space not only plugged into Christian salvation, it
also followed a peculiar late-twentieth-century, middle-class obsession
with safety. Safety as an ethos involved equating the reduction of "risk"
with moral goodness.[52] From suburban neighborhoods to automobiles,
safety was inscribed into the built environment with alarm systems, car
seats, air bags, streetlights, and neighborhood watches. Even shopping
malls linked their success to an ability to furnish safe environs for middle-class female customers.[53] Affluence was made manifest by the level
of security one could achieve, often through isolating middle-class life
from that of "the street." Within this obsession, white women in particu-

lar were trained to constantly monitor their personal safety, which was threatened by a dangerous, often racialized, outside. Gender and privilege, then, further produced the peculiar place of "safety" in the MCS movement. While soldiers with Gulf War syndrome argued before Congressional committees that their claims to illness were all the more "real" because of the contexts of danger and pain that they habitually endured without protest, and while "safe sex" was invoked as a means to rein in promiscuity, the MCS movement's search for safe space was an extension of a gendered and privileged relationship to American "risk" culture.[54]

Though quests for safe space fed into middle-class isolationism, the attraction of a safe space was its ability to displace the site of disability from the body into the environment. Through this attention to space the structures and objects of the built environment became what rendered bodies abled or disabled, healthy or sick. By calling on a familiar gendered performance of house care, and thereby changing the material composition of the built environment, the body could be rendered able again, and rebellious reactions could be tamed. Pathology came to reside in the built environs, not the person.

Bacteria, Information Sharing, and Cyberspace

Scattered around the country, isolated in homes and trailers, MCSers found another safe space in which they could gather in—the newly generated computer-mediated terrain of the Internet. The Internet was safe in three ways. First, it was disembodied and thus able to connect individuals regardless of their physical limitations or "individual biochemistries." Second, it was a supportive space in which people invested in the legitimacy of each other's suffering. Third, within cyberspace one could securely present one's subjectivity; the written format of Internet lists allowed one to respond slowly, without time pressure, helping mentally ill or easily fatigued people who had difficulty with face-to-face interactions participate in social exchange. The production and popularization of the Internet connected people dispersed across distance and individualized isolation and thus made the MCS movement as such possible.

One of the longest running MCS online communities, founded in 1990, was the "Immune" group, which in the middle of the decade was composed of around five hundred participants who called themselves

"Immuners."[55] There was also an active MCS-CI list, and there remains an MCS-Immune-Neuro list, which was described as "a support/information/positive action list to help those with chemical injury and resulting immune and/or nervous system problems manage their illness and lead fulfilling lives."[56] There is even a list called Disinissues, which specialized in disabilities and insurance issues for people with controversial nonspecific illnesses. In cyberspace MCSers found support groups, homepages, and "do-it-yourself" popular culture: people shared information on how to make their own personal ecologies, where to find a "safe" home, do-it-yourself treatments, and therapies that worked for them and might work for others. They offered each other advice and warnings about navigating the workers' compensation machine and other institutional apparatuses, as well as prayers for sustaining the spirit. The Internet was a vital site where MCSers communicated how to grapple with the everyday, a space facilitated by an ethic of information exchange.

One Immuner, aptly tying together cyberspace, the ethic of information exchange, and microbial ecologies, compared the MCS movement to bacteria:

> Part of what makes bacteria so competent as a group and individually is that they have the outstanding quality of SHARING INFORMATION, and cross pollinating different strains of bacteria with this information, so bacteria become much SMARTER and learn how to resist their extermination with antibiotics. In that respect they're sort of like the Borg. We humans could learn a lot from bacteria—it's good we're sharing information on the IMMUNE list![57]

Like bacteria, the MCS movement was cellular and mutable, linked by information exchange online. MCSers came to understand that they had to share information and together "learn how to resist" the constantly changing inside of late capitalism.

Mutations and Body Ecologies

Bodies and the built environment were in a mutual embrace: Where did one end and the other begin? If the personal ecosystem extended to all the objects in a home, why should it stop at our skins? And "why should our bodies end at the skin?"[58] The model of ecosystem management was a useful means of materializing bodies in their environment: its power rested in its ability to absorb objects across scales and domains in terms of, rather than despite, the contingencies of their connections. For MCSers, the body itself was materialized as an individual body-ecology that coped with a potentially manageable personal ecosystem and a dangerous and chaotic late-capitalist out-there. Accordingly, bodies were understood to be so intimately tied to the environment that every symptom could be interpreted as a reaction to the constantly shifting nexus of body-building-ecology. Here, in the encounter between sick bodies and environments, I found "ecology," not simply moving from nature to a corporeal scale but extending from the built environment through the skin, such that the body-ecology and the building-ecology materially intermingled.

For MCSers, the grappling of bodies and the built environment was not just a physical contact between flesh and object but also a molecular interpenetration invisible to the eye. Immune systems and ecosystems bypassed the skin as the ultimate bounds of the body, connecting at the molecular level. Through digestion, respiration, or the epidermis, intermingling resided in the microscopic dimension: antibodies and pollen, T cells and bacteria, chemicals and enzymes. MCSers experimented with populating their body-ecologies with an astounding array of microobjects, each of which required developing a regime of care that could detect and then manipulate it. In particular, MCSers have mobilized molecular technoscientific artifacts in an attempt to get back their intelligibility to biomedicine. Yet they also pulled these technoscientific objects into new associations, spawning new assemblages with which they could cultivate "elsewheres within here."

Immune systems were important artifacts in such body-ecologies.[59] The late-twentieth-century immune system, unlike organs that have precise functions and locations, was everywhere and nowhere in particular. Immune systems, then, were not simply the addition of another organ system, but corporeality at another dimension. They were composed of macrophages, T cells, B cells, and lymphocytes feeding on the microbes that coexisted in bodies, forming a vicious molecular struggle of eat-or-be-eaten. The immune system, not the skin, became the primary delimitation between self and not-self.[60] For MCSers, coping with body-ecologies largely took place at this limit.

Many MCSers also monitored a "detoxification system" that operated in parallel with the immune system, ridding the body of foreign chemicals. The detoxification system has become a crucial part of the body-terrain in the field of clinical ecology. Sherry Rogers, a New York clinical ecologist who has written several popular books, described this body-terrain as "the janitorial service of the body." The detoxification system "keeps it clean so accumulated chemicals do not destroy the machinery."[61] Like the immune system, it is everywhere and nowhere in particular, primarily composed of enzymes that break down chemicals in the body.

The microscopic ecology of the body extended through the organ-filled "body-machine," the immune system, and the detoxification system to include the microbial flora and fauna inhabiting inner spaces. In the body-ecology, humanity's place on the food chain was not clear, as one MCSer explained:

> I think that science has enjoyed placing man at the top of the food chain, King of the ecosphere so to speak, but in actuality, there is one force mightier than us on this planet in every aspect. They are genetically superior, they are far more adaptable, they clearly outnumber us, and they make far better use of their environment—those wee little creatures that von Leeuwenhoek saw through his primitive microscope. They not only facilitate our survival, they also feed on us (maybe Nature's cruel joke is that we are being farmed by microbes?). They are the organisms that truly rule this planet. They started life on this planet and will likely end it (certainly ours is in question). They complete the cycle of life and death that so characterizes nature on every level. (there's even more of their cells than our own in our own bodies!)[62]

This densely populated microbial inner space became another site for intervention. The management of the microbial "ecosphere" could involve extremely complicated and delicate regimes that drew on incredibly detailed knowledge of the body-ecology. Managing overpopulations of the yeast *Candida* was particularly popular. Many recipes and procedures were available at alternative health stores for orchestrating yeast "die off." One MCSer described her method in the following way:

> The Caprylic Acid is fugicidal for both the mycelial form as well as the yeast form of the candida and is harmless to friendly intestinal flora. The Oleic Acid hinders the conversion of the yeast form to the mycelial form. The Psyllium powder forms the gel in the intestinal tract that releases the

Caprylic and Oleic Acids gradually over a period of time and binds them so that they are not sent directly to the liver but stay in the intestinal tract where they are needed.

Additionally, the Psyllium powder scrapes away fecal encrustations that harbor hidden candida, absorbs toxins within the colon, and carries them out. Thus reducing die off symptoms from the toxins of dying candida.

The Bentonite directly absorbs the Candida organisms as well, flushes them out, and absorbs toxins, bacteria, and viruses. By virtue of its physical action, bentonite serves as an adsorbent aid in detoxification of the intestinal canal and is itself not adsorbed by the body. What ever it adsorbs is removed in the feces.

I have to tell you all that this has by far been the easiest die off I have ever experienced.[63]

Within the body ecology, microbial life was not protected like endangered wildlife. Rather, as in a National Park or a building-ecology, the interactions of organisms were managed through sometimes drastic interventions.

None of these objects—т cells, enzymes, or yeast—were simply technoscientific objects of biomedicine; they were artifacts that had been imported into everyday life through techniques for caring for the self, such that мсsers apprehended sickness and health according to the strength or weakness of their immunological, molecular, and microbial ecology. Body-ecologies were difficult to comprehend and control. They did not neatly map onto the biomedical organ systems; they were not simply the addition of an immune system or "detoxification system" onto an older map of the body. The мсs body was materialized as an "elsewhere" organized according to ecological principles precisely because the connections in it could be made to cut across this body map and were constantly adjusting to environmental input.

The dimensions of this body-ecology were not confined to technoscientific or even physical objects: мсsers sometimes evoked spiritual dimensions of their body-ecologies. Christian мсsers made clear what many others believed: the personal ecosystem was composed of not just the physical objects that impinge on the body but also the psychic impingements of traumatic events, stress, and loss of faith. The Alpha Omega Christian Community, for example, explained the cause of мсs as a spiritual wounding of the immune system: "Most of our immune system is formed in our bone marrow. If some event in a person's life wounded their spirit, the person's immune system will have trouble functioning. This is not to say that the cause of disease is psychological. It isn't. The root cause of many diseases is spiritual and that is why doctors have been unable to find a cure for many diseases."[64] For other MCSers, the ecosystem of total impingements included emotional states, stress, and child abuse.

What objects to include in the body-ecology was a contentious issue in the MCS movement. Associating MCS with mental illness was fraught because it evoked the broader stigmatization of mental illness and the specific dematerializing effects of psychosomatic diagnoses. Nonetheless, many MCSers included mental states, particularly depression, in descriptions of their bodily reactions. On Internet support groups, mind-body threads periodically arose where MCSers discussed their different opinions on what influence mental illness, stress, and child abuse had had on their illnesses. In these conversations, mental illness was often biologized as part of brain biochemistry: imbalances in the body-ecology could affect brain chemistry, while emotional states were also chemical states that in turn impacted the rest of the body.[65]

All these objects complexly populating body-ecologies were detected for the purpose of deciphering and influencing ecologies. Body-ecologies were sites for the practice of a do-it-yourself coping. Coping required historically contingent ways of "listening" and intervening. Coping regimes had to be just as individual as body-ecologies. Coping was a technology of the self that necessitated the performance of experiments for cultivating wellness. Coping, as a practice of experimentation, required drawing on and mutating dominant assemblages, sharing information, and pulling objects out of one arrangement and into another.

How to Build Yourself a Body in a Safe Space

Diet, vitamins, algae, saunas, exercise, and detoxing programs all were likely elements of a regime for taming an unruly body with MCS. Women were particularly well-prepared for the experiments necessary to generate such a regime; most had been trained to monitor their own bodies and health through breast self-examinations, birth control technologies, menstrual management, and beauty care using such ordinary tools as mirrors, scales, pregnancy tests, feminine hygiene products, tweezers, and shavers. Tied to this self-monitoring was a gendering of seeking out health care; women were trained to go to their yearly gynecological exam or mammogram and to attend their monthly prenatal visits. In general they were more likely to seek medical care than men. Further, white women, who made up the bulk of MCSers, were more likely to "medicalize" their health.[66] Finally, the intimate work of caretaking—nursing, teaching, and mothering—was gendered. The micromanagement of the body, then, was not a new practice for women with MCS; they called on already available caretaking performances and reconfigured them. Gendered body care usually conducted with cosmetics and weight-loss programs was harnessed and turned to a new end.[67]

Within these MCS coping regimes, symptoms were not the signs of an underlying disease hidden within the body. Instead, symptoms provided MCSers with material information about the way various dimensions of their body-ecologies were interacting. Symptoms were as much indicators of what was going on in the environment as they were indicators of health. Symptoms were not the expression of a disease within; they were both the medium and the message of the body-ecology. They were simultaneously the objects that made up an ecology and signs as to what connections were being made between objects at that moment. Which objects one included in the micromanagement of a body-ecology was contingent on how one "listened" to one's body; what listening devices employed—lab tests, psychological tests, and SPECT scans or prayer, taste, and crystals—shaped what symptoms became audible. Symptoms were information. They were material signs of an interconnection occurring within the ecology. The objects that composed the ecology were in constant communication with each other:

> The human body is more than a mere collection of 50 trillion individual cells because our cells work together. Working together requires coordination, which requires communication. Nerves are just one avenue of communication—the one employed for rapid, discrete messages, such as a quick instruction to a hand, to move away from a hot stove. A large part of the body's internal communication and control is carried out via the bloodstream, where hormones and other chemical messengers move about, carrying signals that not only govern sex and reproduction but also coordinate organs and tissues that work together to keep the body functioning properly.[68]

The microscopic objects within the ecology were apprehended as messengers communicating across scales and dimensions: the medium is the message. MCSers had to learn to listen in on the traffic of information within.

Learning to build yourself a body in a safe space required cautious experimentation.[69] Keep in mind that MCSers were not the only ones experimenting on their bodies. In late-capitalist American culture, many consumers experimented with their bodies to some degree as they tinkered with micromanagement regimes. Some experiments were better mapped than others, and even could be packaged into consumer kits and eventually coded as conformity. When one became sick in an unintelligible manner, experimentation on the body became necessary, and MCSers were compelled to venture into uncharted domains that could spawn unexpected and even dire consequences. Building yourself a body in a safe space required great care.

Here's how.

Pay careful attention because signs can be very subtle and transient. Your body is filled with messages both inconspicuous and debilitating in kind. Learn new ways to listen to how your body feels, how it works, how it connects to the environment. Here's some advice: "I have spent all my savings chasing after all kinds of cures and the best thing I've learned is just to listen to my body."[70] Be meticulous and take care—messages may only be a whisper.

Ecologies have "biochemical individuality," making it necessary to experiment with many listening devices before you can adequately monitor your own. Other MCSers can still be very helpful. Exchanging techniques and advice is an important element in experimentation. Information exchange is the primary ethos of the MCS movement, generating a nationwide exchange circuit in cyberspace. Try listening to what others have already heard. Compare the results:

> Is your tingling in your lips, facial area? A rather strange tingling in my lips is usually one of the first symptoms I have that alerts me that I am beginning to react to something and need to take action to protect myself.[71]

> Sometimes my whole face just feels numb as if it were full of Novocain. Usually the lips and odd taste/tongue sensations precede any odor. At work I pop up from my cubicle like a prairie dog and look around to see who is spraying what.[72]

My tongue gets white looking, tingles and gets jagged edges to it that we call my "dragon tongue." This will happen even when I don't realize I have gotten into something so it is one of my "indicators" of trouble.[73]

In a body-ecology, tingles, numbness, and funny-feeling tongues are not signs that reveal the underlying "disease"; symptoms are signals, information that can help the MCSer plug into how her individual body is grappling with the environment. These signals then suggest how she should intervene in her body-ecology.

Eventually, you will become an expert on your body's rebellions.[74] "The people who know the most about an illness or condition are the people who have it. They may not know it by all its technical names but they know how it looks and feels and what has worked and not worked."[75] You will have to teach your doctor about how your body works. Try and be patient. Most doctors are trained to apprehend symptoms as signs of an internal disease entity codifiable by a medical nosology that, in turn, is captured by linear cause and effect ways of connecting bodies with the world. When you describe your symptoms, biomedicine will likely find them too numerous to correspond to any known disease, too subtle to count as illness in themselves. Paradoxically, it is this plethora of minor complaints that led biomedicine to conclude that MCS was psychosomatic.

Expertise comes slowly, often through years of experimentation, grabbing objects, pulling on lines, inventing new listening devices. As one self-taught expert explained,

I can no longer afford to live with my head in the sand. As things stand today, I have had to learn to be my own best friend, my own best chemist, my own best pharmacist and my own best physician, my own best environmental control engineer. If I had not done that I would be 6 feet under. Living with a chronic illness is not an easy thing as we all know. But we need to be responsible to ourselves and each of us needs to do what our bodies tell us is best for us.[76]

Though you may only become an expert reluctantly, out of necessity, your experiments will generate a rematerialization of your body. Though "listening" is a way to map your illness, to get back onto assemblages, to make sense, it is also a site for materializing a staggeringly detailed and innovative awareness of the body outside of the biomedically intelligible. Through listening, technoscientific molecular objects are absorbed, combined with spiritual elements, and tended with gendered practices.

Through listening, the built environment and the body become intimately linked and interdependent. Keep listening, keep experimenting,
keep pulling on lines and climbing into cells. Take care, care of the self,
but also take heed of the dangers.

Experimentation is dangerous and requires caution. Listening can
turn into an obsession in which every gurgle and crackle resonates with
profound meaning. The connections you form can turn into a net of
lines in which you are caught. While making sense to yourself, you can
quickly become strange and unintelligible to others. Non-mcsers do not
often want to hear your litany of subtle symptoms, and neither do most
doctors. Your quest for a safe space may find you trapped alone in your
home. The gendered performances you draw on may be turned against
you, and you will be seen as just another woman gone mad in a long line
of women gone mad. Obsession can lead to isolation, despair, and black
holes.

Abjection, Materialism, and Multiplicity

Most mcs advocates would likely agree that coping with this relatively
uncharted illness required this kind of personal experimentation.
mcsers would also have been just as likely to affirm a predetermined
reality for mcs revealed by these experiments and, further, to critique
biomedicine for its failure to recognize this reality. Though mcsers may
have been compelled by their circumstances to experiment, that did not
prevent them from wishing that biomedicine would capture mcs, make
sense of it and undo abjection. In the meantime, mcsers have had no
qualms pulling biomedical objects—enzymes, immune systems, lab
tests—into their practices. Within the mcs movement a yearning to fit
into biomedical intelligibility sat next to a critique of biomedicine's ability to determine what bodily states are possible and impossible. How
might historians approach this incongruity?

The favored methodological stance of contemporary social science—
social construction—makes it unsymmetrical, and even hypocritical, to
affirm the reality of abjected bodily conditions uncritically while insist-
ing on the historical contingency of biomedicine. Is there another kind
of political gesture to be made with our methodological toolbox? Or,
does the toolbox itself need changing? That biomedicine is a historically

produced practice, of course, does not negate its successes in manipulating bodies, rendering them intelligible, and easing their suffering. Yet, the strength of historicization has been its ability to demonstrate that this success does not make biomedicine any less historically contingent —the nature of nature has been otherwise, and will be otherwise again. Environmental illness is a concrete example of bodies materialized "otherwise." If we grant that biomedicine materialized bodies, providing helpful ways to perceive them, concrete ways of manipulating them, and tools for inhabiting them, then why should we not grant the same possibility of material effects and capacities to other cultural intelligibilities that coexisted or even conflicted with biomedicine? To point this out is not to argue that the MCS movement did a better or even equal job at materializing bodies, or that all kinds of knowledge should be treated as relative and equivalent. It is to say that the MCS movement made possible a different materialization of bodies and chemical exposure that its practitioners found useful and which made coping possible. It is also to point out that "otherwises" are not relegated to times far in the past but are present in the here and now, in elsewheres within here.

What I have striven to argue through my account of "how to build yourself a body in a safe space" is that abjected illnesses—illnesses marked as impossibilities by biomedicine or the law—could still be made to matter, quite literally, by virtue of practices of caring that connected bodies to the world and allowed suffering to be diminished. Historicity is not inversely proportional to reality—as those who shored up the abjection of MCS have tended to suggest. Nor is abjection absolute. While forging a means for historicizing both MCS and its abjection, I have found it politically necessary to be a materialist who understands matter as the effect of tools, practices, and power, even when exercised at the micro-level of the everyday. The MCS movement did not just create an *explanation* for MCS, it built body-ecologies that were concrete and valuable ways of inhabiting the world.

A more generous and accurate look at biomedicine than the one in this chapter would find, not just a single assemblage, but many different ways of apprehending bodies related to different specialties and subcultures, not to mention dramatically shifting equipment and practices. And conversely, the cells within the MCS movement—such as clinical ecology or cyberspace—are building their own methods that cut up what is perceptible and imperceptible. However, in an uneven world, some ways of perceiving inevitably overshadow others, and some ways just work better, more consistently, and are useful to a wider range of actors. In questions of environmental health, however, when the toxic effect of the vast majority of synthetic chemicals remained untested, when exposures themselves regularly escaped detection, people who believed their bodies were reacting to the background noise of everyday chemicals had very little secure knowledge from which to begin coping with their afflictions. When ignorance has been generated not just accidentally but also purposely—as this book has argued was the case of low-level chemical exposures—then the struggle by ordinary people to understand their bodies and the consequential, sometimes deliberate, undermining of their effort resonates with a political, and not just poignant, valence.

In this book I have tried to juxtapose the practices of professionals and experts such as architects, engineers, corporate and government scientists, business managers, and ecologists with the knowledge-making practices of nonprofessionals such as office workers, feminists, social activists, and MCSers in a way that interrogates the limits through which each brought into perception the background presence of chemical exposures in the late twentieth century. I have tried to treat each of these traditions with equal seriousness but not grant them equal effects in a distinctly uneven world. And it is this unevenness that troubles any easy account of understanding conflicting accounts of environmental harms. The making of office buildings, homes, and other seemingly innocuous places into sites where chemical exposures occurred or did not occur was among other things an effect of power, power that could only be exercised on an uneven terrain.

Life occurred inside. For the city dweller or suburbanite, for the bulk of U.S. citizens at the end of the millennium and into the new, the dramas and banalities of the everyday overwhelmingly occurred within the confines of the built environment. The walls of mechanically ventilated homes, malls, and offices bounded daily life. Sealed, carpeted, and conditioned glittering boxes became the quintessential late capitalist workplaces. The landscape of affluence and privilege that made up much, but not all, of America was a built environment like no other that had ever existed. The tight division between inside and outside made sweating gauche. The solvents that held together the walls, furniture, and cars of material affluence were in their historical infancy. Privilege in postwar America took a form of synthetic opulence never before witnessed.

This new built environment spawned consequences. Bodies were assaulted with detritus and effluent, particulate and molecular dangers. Doorknobs passed bacteria and cars spewed exhaust. Dust mites thrived in carpets, consumed the skin flakes off bodies, and we in turn inhaled their excreta. Pesticides suppressed the vermin indoors as much as on the farm. The chemical plumes and wastes of factories and utilities that huddled at the outskirts of urban grids seeped inside unannounced thanks to modern plumbing. All around, objects emitted odorous or, worse, odorless molecules. Yet in delimited spaces, the chaos was seemingly contained. Air fresheners plugged into sockets. The inside was so often pleasant, affluent, and, orderly.

At stake in the histories this book juxtaposes is our ability not only to notice but also to do something about the health effects of chemical exposures. While this book has been concerned with the background of exposure lurking even in unexceptional spaces of relative comfort, the limits to our ability to monitor and alter chemical exposures apply even more to acuter environmental hazards that are unevenly distributed among disenfranchised people. By tracing a confluence of different material, social, and technical histories, I have tried to demonstrate that the imperceptibility and uncertainty of such harms can be the tangible, and even purposeful, result of human action. When it comes to environmental issues, uncertainty, and thus inaction, is too regularly the purposeful product of state and corporate efforts.

Technically, we could track chemical exposures in other ways, and it has taken effort to make sure that resources are not dedicated to such possibilities. Indeed, even now there could be "personal monitors" that measure accumulated daily exposure to a range of molecules, as were worn by research subjects in the Total Exposure Assessment Methodology studies of 1979.[1] And children could play with pet robot dogs with similar sensors, programmed to detect the presence of volatile organic compounds.[2] And the state could measure, as it does in Sweden, what is called the "total body burden" of accumulated industrial chemicals found in fat and breast milk and regulate the production of chemicals accordingly.[3] And toxicologists could attend to the many different shapes of dose-response curves, recognizing that some chemicals provoke stronger reactions at low levels than at high ones.[4] And scientists could develop new standards of testing that ask how multiple exposures change the level of reaction.[5] And even more basic, peer-reviewed tests could be conducted on the health effects of the tens of thousands of manufactured chemicals now used, but for which no studies exist. And state scientists could simply proceed in their work unhindered and unharrassed. There are many more *and*s to encourage, even as I write this, and as you read this, and now again as this book gathers dust on the shelf. There are many *and*s that you could make that I have neglected. *And. . . . And . . . And . . .*

Introduction

1. Feminist science studies scholarship, of which this book is an example, has made important contributions to our understanding of the history of knowledge and science by focusing on how knowledge is created by a wide range of actors—not just white male experts. The works of scholars such as Adele Clarke, Ruth Schwartz Cowan, Rayna Rapp, and many others have set new standards of analysis that attend to the roles a wide range of nonexpert human actors play in knowledge production and biomedical practice. The sociology of environmental health has also emphasized the importance of knowledge practices from below, as is discussed more fully in chap. 4.

2. See, e.g., Tomes, *Gospel of Germs*.

3. There were many "nonspecific" illnesses, or syndromes, that emerged in the late twentieth century. Despite, or perhaps because of, their proliferation, they are usually controversial. All have in common either a lack of identifiable cause or a diversity of expression, or both. In addition to sick building syndrome and multiple chemical sensitivity, nonspecific illnesses include Gulf War syndrome, chronic fatigue syndrome, acquired immunodeficiency syndrome, cumulative trauma disorder (also called repetitive strain injury), and a host of psychological disorders.

4. I have appropriated the term *materialize* from Judith Butler, who wrote, "What I propose in the place of these conceptions of construction is a return to the notion of matter, not as a site or surface, but as a process of materialization that stabilizes over time to produce the effect of boundary, fixity, and surface we call matter. That matter is always materialized has, I think, to be thought in relation to the productive and, indeed, materializing effects of regulatory power in the Foucaultian sense"; Butler, *Bodies That Matter*, 9–10. Reading Foucault as a materialist, as I also do, Butler describes materiality as an effect of power (2). However, in the bulk of her analyses Butler is primarily concerned with the materialization that occurs through the performativity of language. See, e.g., Butler, "Performativity's Social Magic." In this book I depict materialization as the effect of power as exercised through the concrete arrangements of objects, actions, and subjects, rather than emphasizing the realm of the discursive.

5. *Historical ontology*, as Ian Hacking points out in his book of that title, is a term used by Michel Foucault in his essay, "What Is Enlightenment?," though Foucault himself does not go on to make much use of the term. Much of the strand of scholarship on science concerned with historical ontology is intellectually indebted in some way to Foucault. The scholarship on how objects or phenomena come to exist has also been significantly shaped by the work of Bruno Latour and the actor network theory method of science studies that he influenced. Also important has been the work of historian Lorraine Daston. See Latour, *Pasteurization of France*; and Daston, "Coming into Being of Scientific Objects."

6. Historical ontology builds on historical epistemology. Scholars concerned with historical epistemology examine the historical formation of knowledge production. Scholars also concerned with how objects and their effects come to exist take up questions of historical ontology as well. On this difference, see Hacking, *Historical Ontology*. I use the term *apprehended* purposefully to indicate both the sense of knowing and of a physical capture.

7. For other works that emphasize the multiplicity of objects and ontologies, see Law and Mol, "Notes on Materiality and Sociality"; Law and Mol, *Complexities*; Locke, *Twice Dead*; Mol, *Body Multiple*; and Verran, *Science and an African Logic*.

8. There is a long tradition in science studies of looking at disagreements between different disciplines or scientists. While attending to both the winners and losers in a disagreement, this strand of scholarship has tended to look at how controversies were resolved by one side that successfully defined the terms of valid knowledge. For a classic work in this vein, see Shapin and Schaffer, *Leviathan and the Air-Pump*. Other work has focused on how encounters between different disciplines in collaborative ventures can be productive. See, e.g., Clarke, *Disciplining Reproduction*; and Galison, *Image and Logic*.

9. For an overview of this literature as it relates to environmental health, see Mitman, Murphy, and Sellers, "Cloud over History."

10. See, e.g., Kim Fortun, *Advocacy after Bhopal*; Kirsch, "Harold Knapp"; Nash, "Fruits of Ill-Health"; Petryna, *Life Exposed*; and Luise White, "Poisoned Food."

11. On the history of perception and imperception in modern Europe, see Crary, *Suspensions of Perception*. On the history of ignorance, see Robert Proctor's forthcoming work on agnatology.

12. By using the concept of domains of imperceptibility I do not pretend to be able to capture the radical outside of knowledge. However, I do want to argue that if we identify something as outside, as imperceptible, as unknowable, that something is materialized to some small degree and is thus not radically outside.

13. For an elaboration on this concept, see chap. 1.

14. *Multiplicity* is a concept I have taken from Brian Massumi's English translation of the work of Gilles Deleuze and Félix Guattari. One of the most interesting and useful aspects of multiplicity is the way it displaces difference from within objects and instead posits multiplicity as running through and connecting objects; Deleuze and Guattari, *Thousand Plateaus*, 8. I find their concept of multiplicity a useful way of amending my largely Foucaultian analytic toolbox by allowing me to attend to the encounter between different epistemes and how objects are constituted in such encounters. While I have used several concepts from the work of Deleuze and Guattari to formulate the methodology for this book, my argument here differs substantially from much of the current scholarship in Deleuze studies. Many Deleuze scholars interested in science have followed Deleuze's lead and used scientific and mathematical concepts to formulate their own philosophies of ontology. This book, in contrast, seeks to historicize science and seeks to contribute to analytic approaches in science studies, environmental history, the history of health, and the history of knowledge production.

15. Brian Massumi wrote a wonderful discussion of *and* in his "user's guide" to *A Thousand Plateaus* that describes the *and* in relation to a brick. Massumi, *User's Guide*, 6.

16. Deleuze and Guattari use the excellent example of the wasp and the orchid to describe how two objects materialize each other (though they use the terms "territorialize" or "become"). Deleuze and Guattari, *Thousand Plateaus*, 10. For another example of mutual capture, see Massumi's opening description of the meeting of wood and the woodworker in Massumi, *User's Guide*.

17. Instead of using Foucault's term *discursive formations*, I prefer to use the term *assemblage* from Deleuze and Guattari to emphasize the material culture of formations. Foucault, *Archaeology of Knowledge*, 38. However, "assemblage" is a very complicated part of Deleuze and Guattari's philosophy, and I have appropriated the term and simplified it to my own ends. I prefer it because of its materialist implications: assemblages are formed of not only words, but also objects, actions, and subjects. Foucault also saw "rules of formation" as setting the conditions of existence in a discipline's discourse. For Foucault, rules of formation gave shape to the self-evidencies at work in arrangements of subjects, words, and practices. See ibid. Deleuze and Guattari, building on Foucault, used *assemblage* to describe how words and objects ordered each other and made each other possible according to an "abstract diagram." See Deleuze and Guattari, *Thousand Plateaus*, 503–5.

18. The verb *articulate* is useful because it refers not only to speech, but also to physicality, such as the way the joint articulates an arm.

19. I use *historical regularities* in a Foucauldian sense to mean the abstract

condition of possibility for what was sayable and perceivable in a particular historical circumstance. For example, in vol. I of *The History of Sexuality*, Foucault argues that the Victorian period was characterized not by the repression of sex (which is what one might conclude if one took words literally) but by a proliferation of discussions of sex; it "was taken charge of, tracked down as it were, by a discourse that aimed to allow it no obscurity, no respite"; *History of Sexuality*, 20. Cracking open this discourse, Foucault argues that in fact the condition of possibility for speaking about sex was to explain it as a secret. Regularities, then, are abstracted functions—object functions, subject functions, discursive functions—that set the limits of materialization. What I am trying to get at by "cracking open" is an abstraction, a map of functions or conditions of possibility, not a description of empirical specificities. Deleuze explains this "cracking open" in Deleuze, *Foucault*.

20. Foucault says something similar in his discussion of the "formation of objects": "One cannot speak of anything at any time; it is not easy to say something new; it is not enough for us to open our eyes, to pay attention, or to be aware, for new objects suddenly to light up and emerge out of the ground. But this difficulty is not only a negative one; it must not be attached to some obstacle whose power appears to be, exclusively, to blind, to hinder, to prevent discovery, to conceal the purity of the evidence or the dumb obstinacy of the things themselves; the object does not await in limbo the order that will free it and enable it to become embodied in a visible and prolix objectivity; it does not pre-exist itself, held back by some obstacle at the first edges of light. It exists under the positive conditions of a complex group of relations"; Foucault, *Archaeology of Knowledge*, 44–45. On the agency of nonhuman actors as theorized within science studies, see Latour, *Pasteurization of France* and "Mixing Humans and Nonhumans."

21. Chap. 3 elaborates on and gives an empirical account of rematerialization.

22. Deleuze and Guattari write of "lines of flight" rather than resistance. I think one of their most useful insights about "lines of flight" is that they are dangerous. Just as they can cut across dominant formations and open up possibilities, they are also reterritorializations, which do not escape and can in fact be dangerous and deadly. This is one of the concluding points of chap. 7 in this book. See Deleuze and Parnet, "Many Politics."

23. Spivak explains my position well: "Deconstruction, whatever it may be, is not most valuably an exposure of error, certainly not other people's error, other people's essentialism. The most serious critique in deconstruction is the critique of things that are extremely useful, things without which we cannot live"; Spivak, "In a Word," 4.

1. Man in a Box

1. Any history of the twentieth-century built environment is indebted to Reyner Banham's *The Architecture of the Well-Tempered Environment* (1969). Though over thirty years old, this remains a landmark piece of scholarship.

2. This was the name of the environmental chamber at the Laboratory of Ventilation and Illumination at Harvard University's School of Public Health.

3. Anemometers measure airflow and psychrometers relative humidity.

4. ASHVE was founded in 1894. For histories of the ASHVE, now ASHRAE, through the 1930s, see Carnsdale, "ASHRAE"; Donaldson, *Heat and Cold*; and Janssen, "V in ASHRAE." There was one lone woman engineer in ASHVE's ventilation labs. She was the first woman in the United States to receive a graduate mechanical engineering degree. She went on to work at Willis Carrier's air-conditioning corporation. In staged photographs of the lab published in the ASHVE proceedings, she can sometimes be spotted assuming the position of the experimental subject. In general, however, white men dominated the engineering profession in the early twentieth century. On the history of modern engineering as a white male profession, see Oldenziel, *Making Technology Masculine*.

5. ASHVE instituted its own laboratory in 1919 at the U.S. Bureau of Mines in Pittsburgh, and ASHVE's transactions contain detailed descriptions of ventilation experiments. On the careers of the committee's most prominent members, see ASHVE Research Technical Advisory Committee, "Recent Advances"; Ingles, *Willis Haviland Carrier*; "Charles-Edward Amory Winslow, 1877–1957"; "Constantine Yaglou, 1896–1960"; and Viseltear, "C.-E. A. Winslow."

6. Carrier, "Committee on Temperature."

7. On the history of air conditioning, see Ackerman, *Cool Comfort*; Cooper, *Air-Conditioning America*.

8. On the history of public health reform in America and the place of ventilation, see James Cassedy, *Charles V. Chapin*; Fee, *Disease and Discovery*; Rosen, "Politics and Public Health"; and Rosenkrantz, *Public Health and the State*.

9. Bates, "President's Remarks," 53.

10. Rush, "Rational Basis for Ventilation," 323.

11. This colloquial, middle-class description of the lower classes has been around since well before the nineteenth century.

12. Jackson, *Crabgrass Frontier*; Lipsitz, *Possessive Investment*.

13. On the anticontagionist vs. contagionist debate, see Ackerknecht, "Anticontagionism"; and Hamlin, "Predisposing Causes." The theory that excess carbon dioxide caused foul air had been disproved in an experiment that was to shape ventilation for half a century. This experiment, most notably conducted in America by Lenard Hill in 1913 and in England by J. S.

Haldane, put people in an uncomfortably hot and humid sealed room with a high carbon dioxide concentration. When the subjects used a tube to breathe fresh oxygen-filled air from outside the room, they felt no relief. And when subjects outside breathed in the "foul air" of the sealed room, they felt no discomfort. Thus, it was concluded that carbon dioxide was not the problem. What seemed to offer relief was putting the air in motion. Haldane, "Influence of High Air Temperature"; Hill et al., "Influence of the Atmosphere."

14. New York State Commission on Ventilation, *Ventilation*. On the work of the commission, see Cooper, *Air-Conditioning America*.

15. On the history of building systems in the early twentieth century, see Henry Cowan, *Science and Building*; and Elliot, *Technics and Architecture*.

16. On the history of suspensions of perception within modernity, see Crary, *Suspensions of Perception*.

17. Rush, "Rational Basis for Ventilation," 323. On the history of the human motor, see Price, "Body and Soul"; Rabinbach, *Human Motor*; and Seltzer, *Bodies and Machines*.

18. The Hawthorne Experiments at Western Electric, excellently explored in Gillespie, *Manufacturing Knowledge*, were famous and exemplary instances of this style of experimentation on the relationship between environment and laboring bodies.

19. On the idea of a statistical norm, see Hacking, *Taming of Chance*; and Porter, *Trust in Numbers*. On the development of standardized physical exams, see Nugent, "Fit for Work."

20. Yaglou, Riley, and Coggins, "Ventilation Requirements."

21. Ibid., 134.

22. On the history of this standard, see Carnsdale, "ASHRAE."

23. White-Rogers, advertisement, *ASHRAE Journal* (Jan. 1959).

24. Honeywell, advertisement, *ASHRAE Journal* (Oct. 1963).

25. Milgrome, *Adventure Book of Weather*.

26. Carnsdale, "KSU Emphasizes Applied Research."

27. Banham, *Theory and Design*; Collins, *Changing Ideals*. Philip Johnson and Henry Russel Hitchcock defined the "International Style" of modernist architecture at an exhibit at New York's Museum of Modern Art in 1932. Johnson and Hitchcock, *International Style*. On the relation between Bauhaus and science, see Galison, "Aufbau/Bauhaus."

28. Le Corbusier, *Précisions*, 64ff, quoted in Banham, *Architecture*, 159. The universalizing tendency of this machine aesthetic can also be seen in the following statement also by Le Corbusier: "The buildings of Russia, Paris, Suez, or Buenos Aires, the steamer crossing the equator, will be hermetically closed—in winter warmed, in summer cooled—which means that pure, controlled air at 18 degrees Celsius circulates within forever" (ibid.).

29. Jordy, "Aftermath of the Bauhaus." Despite its application of a functionalist aesthetic, the Bauhaus school of architecture was subsequently criticized for just having a functional look and not being truly concerned with a functional use.

30. SOM is perhaps best known in architecture history for designing Lever House (1952), a Manhattan office building with one of the first all-glass-curtained walls. The landmark, total world, SOM-designed Connecticut General headquarters was completed in 1957. SOM went on to work on office buildings for IBM, Philip Morris, General Electric, United Airlines, American Can, Reynolds Aluminum, Emhart, H. J. Heinz, Upjohn, Boise Cascade, and Weyerhaeuser. For my understanding of corporate architecture, I am indebted to Jeffrey Inaba, "Corporate Office Design."

31. For a great spoof of the corporate machine, watch the wonderful film *The Apartment* (1960), directed by Billy Wilder.

32. Biggs, *Rational Factory.*

33. Whyte, *Organization Man.* The kind of lifestyle and jobs Whyte described fell apart in the 1980s with dramatic layoffs in the managerial class. See Bennett, *Death of Organization Man.* More generally on the professional middle class's representation of itself, see Ehrenreich, *Fear of Falling.*

34. The term comes from Galbraith, *Affluent Society.*

35. For an edifying account of the rules of development, see Garreau, *Edge City.*

36. Propst, *Office,* 29. For more on Propst, see chap. 2.

37. Thompson and McHugh, *Work Organizations*; Waring, *Taylorism Transformed.*

38. In 1972, the utopic "machine for living" took a blow when Pruitt-Igoe in St. Louis, the award-winning housing development inspired by Le Corbusier, was deemed uninhabitable and demolished (a moment Charles Jencks identifies as the beginning of postmodernism). Also see critiques of the Bauhaus school's functionalist aesthetic and the universalism implicit in Banham's important study of the built environment. See Banham, *Architecture*; and Harvey, *Condition of Postmodernity.*

39. ASHRAE standard 62–74. Also, ASHRAE standard 90–75, *Energy Conservation in New Building Design.* The standard 62 was modified again in 1981 and 1989 to differentiate between smoking and nonsmoking spaces.

2. Building Ladies

1. There is a debate about the class status of office workers: Are they part of the middle class or the proletariat? This binary framing of the question is inadequate to the variety of kinds of office work as well as the gender and

race stratifications that inform who is eligible for office work, both as they have changed over time with the opening up of managerial positions to white women and processing positions to women of color and as they change over space, from American urban centers to suburbs to offshore sites in poor regions. One of the main assertions of this chapter is that office work is constituted via this tension about its status.

2. Braverman, *Labor and Monopoly Capital.*

3. In his *Discipline and Punish,* Foucault uses this notion of the apparatus to analyze the prison as a historically specific technology of discipline and subjection. Foucault defines *apparatus* in the following way, "What I am trying to pick out with this term is, firstly, a thoroughly heterogeneous ensemble consisting of discourses, institutions, architectural forms, regulatory decisions, laws, administrative measures, scientific statements, philosophical, moral and philanthropic propositions—in short, *the said as much as the unsaid.* Such are the elements of the apparatus. The apparatus itself is the system of relations that can be established between these elements"; Foucault, *Discipline and Punish,* 145–46; my emphasis. My analysis of the office as an apparatus, however, differs from Foucault's analysis of the prison. Foucault does a marvelous job at drawing his topography in terms of the knowledges and material technologies that maintained subjection, and thus he tended to represent the prisoner as the outcome or effect of the orderly workings of the prison. In chap. 3, I draw a topography of the material technologies of resistance that interfered with and rematerialized the office as described here.

4. This account draws heavily from the many feminist historians who have described the emergence of office work in the late nineteenth century and its subsequent feminization and rationalization in the years before World War II, especially the rich account of the rise of Taylorized office work in Strom, *Beyond the Typewriter.* See also Aron, *Ladies and Gentlemen*; Davies, *Women's Place*; Devault, *Sons and Daughters*; Fine, *Souls of the Skyscraper*; Lupton, *Mechanical Brides*; Massachusetts History Workshop, *They Can't Run the Office*; and Rotella, *Home to Office.*

5. On Taylorism, see Banta, *Taylored Lives*; Braverman, *Labor and Monopoly Capital*; Nelson, *Fredrick W. Taylor*; and Yates, *Control through Communication.*

6. Strom, *Beyond the Typewriter,* 182–83.

7. Light, "When Computers Were Women"; Lapartito, "When Women Were Switches."

8. Davies, *Women's Place.*

9. Green, *Race on the Line.*

10. Leffingwell, *Office Management.*

11. Leffingwell, *Scientific Office Management.* On the application of Taylor-

ism in the office, see Strom's "Managers, Clerks and the Question of Gender," in Strom, *Beyond the Typewriter*, 227–69.

12. Thompson, *Soundscape of Modernity*.

13. Haigh, "Inventing Information Systems."

14. Haigh, "Chromium-Plated Tabulator."

15. Waring, *Taylorism Transformed*.

16. For the history of office furniture and technologies, see Forty, *Objects of Desire*; and Lupton, *Mechanical Brides*.

17. For a description of this building, see Becker and Steele, *Workplace by Design*, 27–28.

18. The trope of the corporate family goes back at least to the progressive era; Kwolek-Folland, *Engendering Business*; Mandell, *Corporation as Family*.

19. Garrison, *Electronic Sweatshop*.

20. Ehrenreich, *Fear of Falling*.

21. Green, *Race on the Line*.

22. Greenbaum, *Windows on the Workplace*.

23. Meikle, *American Plastic*.

24. Wiener, *Use of Human Beings*.

25. For overviews of office layouts in the postwar period, see Delgado, *Enormous File*; Kleeman, *Interior Design of the Electronic Office*; Klein, *Office Book*; Pile, *Open Office Planning*; Pile, *Open Office Space*; and Shoshkes, *Space Planning*.

26. Galison, "Ontology of the Enemy."

27. Pile, *Open Office Planning*, 29–32.

28. On reengineering in general, see Castells, *Rise of Network Society*.

29. For an overview of work organization, see Thompson and McHugh, *Work Organizations*. For an influential model of the flexible firm from the Institute of Manpower Studies, see Atkinson, "Manpower Strategies." On the restructuring of the office in particular, see Greenbaum, *Windows on the Workplace*.

30. Carla Freeman, *High Tech and High Heels*.

31. Grossman, "Women's Place in the Integrated Circuit." See also, Fox, *Toxic Work*; Haraway, "Cyborg Manifesto"; and Ong, *Spirits of Resistance*.

32. For more on the cubicle office, see Greenbaum, *Windows on the Workplace*.

33. Anonymous female VDT operator at a New York newspaper, quoted in Judith Gregory's testimony on behalf of 9to5 in U.S. House Committee on Education and Labor, *New Technology in the American Workplace: Hearings by the Subcommittee of Education and Labor*, June 23, 1982. 9to5 papers, box 5, folder 154.

34. Copeland, *Generation X*.

35. Pulgram and Stonis, *Designing the Automated Office*, 37.

36. Kleeman, *Interior Design of the Electronic Office.*

37. For a description of this new Union Carbide building, see ibid., 213.

38. Donald Nightengale, 1981, quoted in ibid., 214.

39. Gere Picasso, 1985, quoted in ibid., 215.

40. The best account of the history of the Hawthorne experiments is Gillespie, *Manufacturing Knowledge.*

41. On the way computers transformed clerical work in the 1970s and early 1980s, see Barker and Downing, "Word Processing"; Glenn and Feldberg, "Proletarianizing Clerical Work"; Hartmann, *Computer Chips and Papers Clips*; and Nussbaum, "Office Automation."

42. Zuboff, *Age of the Smart Machine.*

43. Jain, "Inscription Fantasies and Interface Erotics."

44. Glenn and Feldberg, "Proletarianizing Clerical Work," 55.

45. Greenbaum, *Windows on the Workplace*, 101.

46. Cunningham and Zalokar, "Economic Progress of Black Women."

47. Braverman, *Labor and Monopoly Capital*, 297.

48. Nussbaum, "Office Automation," 16.

3. Feminism, Surveys, Toxic Details

1. Botsch, *Organizing the Breathless*; Claudia Clark, *Radium Girls*; Judkins, *We Offer Ourselves as Evidence*; Rosner and Markowitz, *Deadly Dust*; Barbara Ellen Smith, *Digging Our Own Graves.*

2. I use "hail" here in relation to Louis Althusser's notion of interpellation and its reworking in terms of performativity by Judith Butler; Althusser, "Ideology and Ideological State Apparatuses," and Butler, *Bodies That Matter.*

3. On microphysics, see Foucault, *History of Sexuality.*

4. This is a paraphrase from Haraway, "Situated Knowledges," 191.

5. Dembe, *Occupation and Disease*; Higgens-Evenson, "Industrial Police."

6. Which diseases to include on these schedules became a contentious issue between workers' and state compensation systems, as expressed in the black and brown lung movements of the 1960s and 1970s. In the 1970s, a federal report critiqued such systems as out of date; National Commission on State Workmen's Compensation Laws, *Report.* State after state amended its laws to include any occupational disease that could be demonstrated to be caused, aggravated, or hastened by the workplace. A worker must still document that he or she is suffering from a particular disease, however, and that this disease is considered by occupational health professionals to be caused by conditions found at their workplace. Though it is technically possible to get compensation for a chronic injury, such as a back injury, the burden of proof is on the worker. Dembe, *Occupation and Disease.*

7. Sellers, *Hazards of the Job.*

8. *Popular epidemiology* was coined in Phil Brown, "Popular Epidemiology." For a detailed history of popular epidemiology as it relates to indoor pollution, see chap. 4.

9. On the relationship between feminism and labor movements, see Bell, "Unionized Women"; Briskin and McDermott, *Women Challenging Unions*; Feldberg, "'Union Fever'"; Goldberg, *Organizing Women*; Kates, "Working Class Feminism"; Sansbury, "'Now What's the Matter?'"; and Seifer and Wertheimer, "New Approaches."

10. This, however, was not the first time women office workers had heard the call of feminism, or even of labor organizing; Feldberg, "'Union Fever'"; Strom, "'We're No Kitty Foyles.'"

11. Jean Tepperman documented the feminist clerical movement in the Boston area. She published two books and interviewed many clerical workers in 1974 and 1975. Tepperman, *Sixty Words a Minute* and *Not Servants.* The interviews are archived at the Schlesinger Archive, Radcliffe College, Harvard University.

12. Susan Davis, "Organizing from Within."

13. Plotke and Nussbaum, "Women Clerical Workers," 153.

14. Ibid., 154–55.

15. Echols, *Daring to Be Bad.*

16. Davidow, "Acting Otherwise," 36–37; Shreve, *Women Together, Alone,* 11.

17. *Women Office Workers News*, Jan.–Feb. 1974.

18. *Women Office Workers News*, April–May 1974.

19. Quoted in Cassedy and Nussbaum, *9 to 5,* 158.

20. The film was used as a vehicle to promote the women office workers' movement. Jane Fonda went on a national promotional tour with it. The movie's success went on to spawn a hit single, Dolly Parton's "Working 9 to 5," and a short-lived television series in 1982.

21. On experience, see Bellamy and Leontis, "Genealogy of Experience"; Mohanty, "Feminist Encounters"; and Scott, "'Experience.'"

22. Sarachild, "Consciousness-Raising," 132.

23. This is not to argue that all feminists were concerned with details rather than with structural inequalities.

24. Herman Miller Office Furniture advertisement, *Wall Street Journal,* Nov. 14, 1974.

25. Karen Nussbaum, quoted in Tepperman, *Not Servants,* 89.

26. Herman Miller Office Furniture advertisement, *Wall Street Journal,* Nov. 14, 1974.

27. It is interesting to note the striking similarity between this analysis and the one developed roughly contemporaneously by Michel Foucault, who

showed how the operation of any modern institutional apparatus, be it a prison or an office, is exercised in the abundance of small details, of daily gestures, bodily disciplines, habits, schedules, spatial demarcations, and repetitions—what he called the "microphysics" of power, or the "capillary" operation of power.

28. 9to5, *Hidden Victims*; 9to5, *VDT Syndrome*; Marschall and Gregory, *Office Automation*; Tepperman, *Sixty Words a Minute*; Tepperman, *Not Servants*; Working Women, *Race against Time*.

29. "Health and Safety: Writing and Negotiating Your Union Contract," *Union WAGE*, March–April 1975.

30. Though there is to date no proof that VDTS are linked to reproductive health problems, concern remains among some activists that low-level radiation may be unhealthy.

31. With a PhD in physical chemistry (1972) from the City University of New York, Stellman began working on occupational health issues with industrial unions. Before the early 1970s, there were very few studies of women and occupational illnesses, and Stellman was part of the vanguard of women in the 1970s who defined this area of study. However, a few famous occupational diseases had affected women, such as the radiation poisoning of radium dial painters and phosphorus poisoning of women who worked in match factories. See Claudia Clark, *Radium Girls*; and Moss, "Kindling a Flame."

32. Women's Occupational Health Resource Center, "Clerical Workers: Fact Sheet," Stellman papers, box 2, unlabelled black folder.

33. Jeanne Stellman, speech, Institute on Safety and Health, Columbus, Ohio; quoted in Banning, "Workplace Chemicals," 16.

34. Photocopiers had been maligned in the press in a series of articles with titles such as "Cancer from Photocopiers?," *Mother Jones*, Dec. 1980, 8; Lofroth et al., "Mutagenic Activity"; and "IBM Brass Knew TNF 'Possible' Carcinogen More than a Decade Ago," *Computerworld*, Sept. 8, 1980, 1.

35. Anita Reber, testimony before the House Committee on Interstate and Foreign Commerce, Subcommittee on Health and the Environment, 97th Congress, 1st sess., Feb. 4, 1981. Also see NIOSH Health Hazard Evaluation Number 76-70-367.

36. Consumer Product Safety Commission, "Alert Sheet."

37. Karen Nussbaum, speech, Women's Occupational Health Resource Center, New York, Oct. 1981. Quoted in "Sending a Letter: PCBS and Other Office Hazards," *Working Women News*, Nov.–Dec. 1981.

38. Stellman and Henifin, *Office Work*, 63.

39. Colligan, "Review of Mass Psychogenic Illness"; Schmitt, Colligan, and Fitzgerald, "Unexplained Physical Symptoms."

40. Susan Davis, "Organizing from Within."

41. In fact, some of the volunteers in Project Health and Safety critiqued the way the organization of the committee reflected office work itself. As one volunteer explained in her resignation letter, "In our questionnaires, we inquired about the issue of lack of control as being a contributory factor causing stress in the workplace. I feel a lack of control and input into committee decisions that is as devastating as that which I currently experience in my workplace. It is as if the decisions for the Committee have already been made by 9to5 and Working Women in advance and we are simply to fulfill these constant requests. The members do not appear to be an integral part of the decision-making process." Letter of resignation to Health and Safety Committee, 9to5 papers, May 6, 1981, box 5, folder 150. The committee was also critiqued for not representing the diversity of office workers (committee members tended to be young, college-educated, white, and single). Self-evaluation of the Committee on Health and Safety, 9to5 papers, July 7, 1981, box 5, folder 151.

42. Gordon, *Pitied but Not Entitled*; Silverberg, *Gender and American Social Science*; Sklar, "Hull-House Maps and Papers."

43. According to the survey, 70% of women clerical workers experienced an inadequate supply of fresh air, two-thirds reported air circulation problems, and 25% reported irritating fumes. Stress was also widely reported, particularly among office workers who used VDTS.

44. For examples of surveys, see Makower, *Office Hazards*; Stellman, *Women's Work*; Stellman and Henifin, *Office Work*; and Working Women, *Warning*.

45. On the history of objectification through quantification, see Galison and Daston, "Image of Objectivity"; Hacking, *Taming of Chance*; and Porter, *Trust in Numbers*.

46. Lisa Fein, "9to5's Project Health and Safety," letter to Rep. T. Moffett, U.S. House of Representatives, April 24, 1981, 9to5 papers, box 5, folder 150.

47. Mary Mitchell, speech, April 22, 1981, 9to5 papers, box 5, folder 150.

48. 9to5, *National Survey*.

49. Singer et al., "Mass Psychogenic Illness." On the history of menstruation and work, see Cayleff, "'She Was Rendered Incapacitated'"; Harlow, "Function and Dysfunction"; Emily Martin, *Woman in the Body*, 92–138; and Walker, "History of Menstrual Psychology."

50. Nussbaum, "Office Automation," 19.

51. "Clerical Workers Tell All," *Union WAGE*, July–Aug. 1979, 3.

52. M. G. Smith, "Potential Health Hazards."

53. Haynes and Feinleib, "Women, Work and Heart Disease."

54. "Stress Is a Social Disease," 1973. Reprinted in *Processed World*, Fall 1987, 41.

55. Selye, *Stress of Life*.

56. Stellman, *Women's Work*, 42.

57. "Stress: The Office Worker's Illness," *9to5 Newsletter*, Sept.–Oct. 1993, 3.

58. Neurasthenia, hysteria, and nerves, like stress, were also thought to result from the "new" anxieties of their moment. Kugelmann, *Stress*.

59. Nussbaum, "Office Automation," 19.

60. Fonda, *Jane Fonda's Workout Book*.

61. In this same period, psychosomatic explanations split into two politically divergent camps. In the first, and more politically conservative, form, physical illness with no known biological underpinning is explained, usually by a process of elimination, as a somatic expression of an underlying, gendered psychological disorder or disposition. In its second, and more politically radical, form, psychosomaticism is understood as a biological expression caused by racial, sexual, or other kinds of oppression. Thus, there is a recent, scientifically rigorous epidemiological literature on the relationship between racism and hypertension. For a historical account of this association, see Greenlee, "Biomedicine and Ideology."

62. Before holding this post, Nussbaum was appointed to head the Women's Bureau of the Labor Department during President Bill Clinton's first term. On the recent increase of women in unions, both in the rank and file and in positions of power, see Kosterlitz, "Luring Women to Labor's Ranks"; and Waldman, "Labor's New Face." This increase in unionism among women has come hand-in-hand with a return to organizing techniques that involve one-to-one contact. See, e.g., Hoerr, *We Can't Eat Prestige*.

63. See, e.g., Boxer, "Occupational Mass Psychogenic Illness"; Colligan, "Psychological Effects"; Faust and Brilliant, "Diagnosis of 'Mass Hysteria'"; and Ryan and Morrow, "Dysfunctional Buildings or Dysfunctional People."

4. Toxicology and Epidemiology

1. Wallingford, *NIOSH IEQ Health Hazard Evaluation Requests*.

2. U.S. House of Representatives, Indoor Air Quality Act of 1990 Report (May 24, 1990), 37.

3. For a detailed account of the CIAR, see Barnes and Biro, "Industry-Funded Research."

4. Wallingford, *NIOSH IEQ Health Hazard Evaluation Requests*.

5. The first published use of the term was in Stolwijk, "Sick Building Syndrome" (1984).

6. See responses to the first mention of the term *SBS* in a major journal; Finnegan, Pickering, and Burge, "Sick Building Syndrome" (1985).

7. The first factory inspections of the late nineteenth century targeted

women and children. Restrictions on phosphorous, benzene, lead, and radium, some of the earliest chemicals regulated by the state, were also enacted in the name of protecting women. Historian Allison Hepler points out that it was only after the 1870s, when courts struck down laws meant to regulate male workers' hours and conditions, that reformers turned their attention to women workers; Hepler, *Women in Labor*.

8. The field of occupational medicine is composed of several different types of experts. The occupational physician is a doctor who specializes in occupational medicine. He or she is trained to identify and treat occupational illnesses and diseases. The industrial hygienist, whose job it is to inspect the health and safety of workplaces, is not typically a physician. Industrial hygienists are experts in the detection of chemicals or hazards in the workplace. They use a different set of tools and do not treat patients but rather search for the causes of occupational illnesses. Reflecting this division, occupational health textbooks are typically ordered by either hazard or organ system.

9. For an overview of the history of chemistry, see Bensaude-Vincent and Stengers, *History of Chemistry*; and Brock, *Norton History of Chemistry*.

10. Occupational medicine emerged much later in the United States than it did in European countries such as England and Germany, where it developed in the nineteenth century.

11. On Alice Hamilton, see Hamilton, *Exploring the Dangerous Traces*; Hepler, *Women in Labor*; and Sicherman, *Alice Hamilton*.

12. That Hamilton was a woman interested in occupational health was not exceptional. On the contrary, in the early twentieth century, women reformers who ran the Consumer League and the Worker's Health Bureau were important actors in focusing political attention on and instigating protective legislation about industrial work conditions.

13. Hepler, *Women in Labor*.

14. Ibid.

15. On the history of surveys, see Bulmer, "Decline of the Social Survey."

16. My account of industrial hygiene in the interwar years borrows heavily from and is indebted to Sellers, *Hazards of the Job*. I urge any reader wanting to know more about industrial hygiene in this time period to consult it. For the literature on the history of occupational disease in the United States, see Bayer, *Health and Safety of Workers*; Berman, "Why Work Kills"; Claudia Clark, *Radium Girls*; Corn, *Protecting the Health of Workers*; Fox, *Toxic Work*; Judkins, *We Offer Ourselves as Evidence*; Nelkin and Brown, *Workers at Risk*; Rosner and Markowitz, *Deadly Dust*; Rosner and Markowitz, *Deceit and Denial*; Rosner and Markowitz, *Dying for Work*; Sellers, "Factory as Environment"; Sheehan and Wedeen, *Toxic Circles*; Barbara Ellen Smith, *Digging Our Own Graves*; and Weindling, *Social History of Occupational Health*.

17. During this period, physical exams were standardized by the insurance industry so that they would both be "efficient"—that is, quickly administered —and create data for statistical comparison. On the history of the physical exam, see Audrey Davis, "Life Insurance"; and Nugent, "Fit for Work."

18. For the source of these arguments and a detailed account of the lab at Harvard see chap. 5, "*Pax Toxicologia*," in Sellers, *Hazards of the Job*, 141–86.

19. Ibid.

20. Lawrence Henderson, "Effects of Social Environment."

21. On lead-poisoning research, see Hepler, *Women in Labor*; Sellers, *Hazards of the Job*; and Warren, *Brushes with Death*.

22. On history of the ACGIH, see Corn, *Protecting the Health of Workers*.

23. Other countries, such as Canada and many European nations continued to use and develop the MAC.

24. See "The Political Morphology of Dose-Response Curves," in Proctor, *Cancer Wars*, 153–73; and Paull, "Origin and Basis of Threshold Limit Values."

25. On the use of animals in occupational health research, see Messing and Mergler, " 'Rat Couldn't Speak.' "

26. The rise of the corporate research lab is nicely documented in a case study of R and D at DuPont. Hounshell and Smith, *Science and Corporate Strategy*.

27. Castleman and Ziem, "Corporate Influence"; Castleman and Ziem, "American Conference"; Markowitz and Rosner, "Limits of Thresholds"; Roach and Rappaport, "But They Are Not Thresholds."

28. Corn, *Protecting the Health of Workers*, 36–37.

29. See Murray, "Regulating Asbestos"; Ozonoff, "Failed Warnings"; Rosner and Markowitz, *Deadly Dust*; and Rosner and Markowitz, *Deceit and Denial*.

30. On the history of workers' compensation, see Bale, " 'Hope in Another Direction,' " parts 1 and 2; Berman, "Why Work Kills"; Boden, "Problems in Occupational Disease Compensation"; Greenwood, "Historical Perspective"; and Higgens-Evenson, "Industrial Police."

31. For example, brown lung, associated with the textile industry, does not show up on X-rays and remains questioned; Judkins, *We Offer Ourselves as Evidence*.

32. The exceptions to this rule in the 1970s and early 1980s were specific cases of asbestos, radon, and formaldehyde poisoning, as well as acute outbreaks of pathogens inside ventilation systems, such as the deadly Legionnaires' disease or humidifier fever.

33. Hicks, "Tight Building Syndrome."

34. The first U.S. study to meet such standards was published in 1983. Researchers in the Lawrence Berkeley Laboratory studied a San Francisco office building, comparing workers' symptoms under two different ventila-

tion rates, a reduced rate and a higher control rate. These epidemiologists concluded that under conditions of reduced ventilation workers' symptoms increase. They claimed that pollutant levels did not "exceed current health standards for outdoor air, nor was any one contaminant found to be responsible. . . . It is possible that a synergistic effect of the various contaminants and environmental conditions may account for the discomfort of occupants"; Turiel et al., "Effects of Reduced Ventilation."

35. Bauer, Greve, et al., "Role of Psychological Factors"; Boxer, "Occupational Mass Psychogenic Illness"; Colligan, "Psychological Effects"; Colligan, "Review of Mass Psychogenic Illness"; Faust and Brilliant, "Diagnosis of 'Mass Hysteria' "; Guitotti, Alexander, and Fedoruk, "Epidemiologic Features"; Kerckhoff and Back, *June Bug*; Rothman and Weintraub, "Sick Building Syndrome and Mass Hysteria"; Ryan and Morrow, "Dysfunctional Buildings or Dysfunctional People"; Schmitt, Colligan, and Fitzgerald, "Unexplained Physical Symptoms"; Stahl and Legedun, "Mystery Gas."

36. Colligan and Murphy, "Mass Psychogenic Illness."

37. Ibid.

38. Boxer, "Occupational Mass Psychogenic Illness."

39. Colligan and Murphy, "Mass Psychogenic Illness."

40. Singer et al., "Mass Psychogenic Illness."

41. Boxer, "Occupational Mass Psychogenic Illness."

42. Colligan and Murphy, "Mass Psychogenic Illness."

43. Phil Brown, "Popular Epidemiology."

44. Allan, *Uneasy Alchemy*; Phil Brown, "Popular Epidemiology"; Brown and Ferguson, " 'Making a Big Stink' "; Brown and Mikkelsen, *No Safe Place*; Bullard, "Environmental Justice for All"; Di Chiro, "Defining Environmental Justice"; Di Chiro, "Local Actions, Global Visions"; Fischer, *Citizens, Experts and the Environment*; Kim Fortun, *Advocacy after Bhopal*; Krauss, "Blue-Collar Women and Toxic-Waste Protests"; Krauss, "Women and Toxic Waste Protests"; Krauss, "Challenging Power."

45. Popular epidemiology was crucial, for example, in identifying incidents of toxic contamination by General Electric of Pittsfield, Mass.; by the Pelham Bay dump in a Bronx, N.Y. neighborhood; by Martin Marietta Corporation in Friendly Hills, Colo.; by Velsicol Chemical Corporation in Hardeman County, Tenn.; and by W. R. Grace and Company and Beatrice Foods in Woburn, Mass.; Brown and Mikkelsen, *No Safe Place*, 127; Frumkin and Kantrowitz, "Cancer Clusters in the Workplace." It has also been important in the environmental justice movement, such as in the attempt to litigate a claim of environmental racism in the Northwood Manor neighborhood of Houston in 1979; Blum, "Pink and Green."

46. The best work on the history of the social survey movement is Bulmer, Bales, and Sklar, *Social Survey*.

47. College Settlements Association, *Fourth Annual Report*, 22–23; quoted in Katz and Sugrue, *W. E. B. DuBois*, 14.

48. Bulmer, "W. E. B. Du Bois"; Katz and Sugrue, *W. E. B. DuBois*.

49. DuBois, *Philadelphia Negro*, 1.

50. Bay, " 'World Was Thinking Wrong.' "

51. DuBois, *Philadelphia Negro*, 8.

52. Ibid.

53. Lasch-Quinn, *Black Neighbors*.

54. Sklar, "Hull-House Maps and Papers."

55. Sinclair-Holbrook, "Map Notes and Comments," 11–12.

56. Ibid., 11.

57. Ibid., 5.

58. On "geographical sentiment" at Hull House, see Sklar, "Hull House Maps and Papers."

59. Kelley, "Hull House," 550.

60. DuBois, *Autobiography*, 198; DuBois, *Philadelphia Negro*, 3.

61. DuBois, *Souls of Black Folk*, 4.

62. Steven Cohen, "Pittsburgh Survey."

63. Bulmer, Bales, and Sklar, "Social Survey," 30.

64. Bulmer, "Decline of the Social Survey."

65. Beck, "Industrial Society to Risk Society."

66. Carson, *Silent Spring*, 168.

67. On popular epidemiology as citizen science, see, Di Chiro, "Local Actions, Global Visions"; and Fischer, *Citizens, Experts and the Environment*.

68. Murphy, "Immodest Witnessing."

69. For an expansive discussion of maternalism in American women's environmental activism, see Blum, "Pink and Green."

70. Zeff, Love, and Stults, *Empowering Ourselves*.

71. Theresa Freeman, "Vermonters Organized," 43.

72. Quoted in Di Chiro, "Defining Environmental Justice," 120.

73. For accounts of Love Canal, see Blum, "Pink and Green"; Fowlkes and Miller, "Chemicals and Community"; Gibbs, *Love Canal*; Levine, *Love Canal*; and Mazur, *Hazardous Inquiry*.

74. Krauss, "Blue-Collar Women and Toxic-Waste Protests"; Lipsitz, *Possessive Investment*.

75. For more on the way racialized distributions of privilege and disadvantage shaped the science of indoor pollution, see chap. 5.

76. On the Newtown Florists Club, see Spears, "Environmental Justice." On the importance of benevolent societies and women's clubs in early African-American women's environmentalism, see Blum, "Pink and Green."

77. Allan, *Uneasy Alchemy*; Rosner and Markowitz, *Deceit and Denial*.

78. Bryant and Mohai, "Environmental Injustice"; Bullard, "Environmen-

tal Justice for All"; General Accounting Office, "Siting of Hazardous Waste Landfills," 83–168; United Church of Christ Commission on Racial Justice, *Toxic Wastes and Race.*

79. Newman, "Killing Legally." Also see Di Chiro, "Defining Environmental Justice."

80. Newman, "Killing Legally."

81. Cohen and O'Connor, *Fighting Toxics*; Environmental Action Foundation, *Making Polluters Pay*; Legator, Harper, and Schott, *Health Detectives Handbook.*

82. Stolwijk, "Sick-Building Syndrome" (1991), 99.

83. U.S. Environmental Protection Agency, "Inside Story," 35.

84. Finnegan and Pickering, "Building Related Illness," 391.

5. Uncertainty, Race, EPA Activism

1. Crary, *Suspensions of Perception.*

2. Important contributions to the study of white privilege in science include Warwick Anderson, "Trespass Speaks"; and Morawski, "White Experimenters."

3. On white privilege, see Delgado and Stefancic, *Critical White Studies*; Lipsitz, *Possessive Investment*; and Rasmussen et al., *Making and Unmaking.*

4. Winant, "White Racial Projects."

5. Dyer, "White," 44.

6. Borchert, *Alley Life.*

7. Gillette, *Between Justice and Beauty.*

8. Diner, "Washington"; Jones, "Before Montgomery and Greensboro."

9. Gilbert, *Ten Blocks*; Kofie, *Race, Class.*

10. U.S. Census, demographic data for zip code 20024 (1990).

11. Lipsitz, *Possessive Investment.*

12. See, e.g., Green, *Race on the Line.*

13. Lipsitz, *Possessive Investment*, 7.

14. In addition to Lipsitz, *Possessive Investment*, see Mahoney, "Residential Segregation"; and Sacks, "G.I. Bill."

15. Lipsitz, *Possessive Investment.*

16. Manning, "Multicultural Washington," 337.

17. U.S. EPA, *Affirmative Program Plan*, 49.

18. Ibid., 52.

19. Krauss, "Challenging Power."

20. Gibbs, *Love Canal*, 12.

21. Patty Fraser, quoted in Zeff, Love, and Stults, *Empowering Ourselves,* 13.

22. For the history of how university industrial hygienists fashioned themselves in this way, see Sellers, *Hazards of the Job.*

23. "The Reagan Effect," in Proctor, *Cancer Wars.*

24. On the history of the EPA during the 1980s, see Land, Roberts, and Thomas, *Environmental Protection Agency*; and Lash, Gillman, and Sheridan, *Season of Spoils.*

25. William Ruckelshaus, interview by Michael Gain, EPA History Office, Washington, D.C., Jan. 1993.

26. Sanjour, "EPA's Revolving Door," 77.

27. Lavelle and Coyle, "Special Investigation."

28. See, e.g., Bryant and Mohai, "Environmental Injustice"; Bullard, *Confronting Environmental Racism*; and General Accounting Office, "Siting of Hazardous Waste Landfills."

29. United Church of Christ Commission on Racial Justice, *Toxic Wastes and Race*, ix–x.

30. On the relationship between environmental justice and the EPA, see Sandweiss, "Social Construction."

31. National Treasury Employees Union (NTEU), Chapter 280, "The Official History of NTEU, Chapter 280: Seventeen Years of Public Service at the EPA," April 9, 2001, http://www.nteu280.org/history.htm (accessed June 14, 2001).

32. In Feb. 1998, members voted to change affiliation from the NFFE to the National Treasury Employees Union, Chapter 280.

33. NTEU, Chapter 280, "Official History."

34. NTEU, Chapter 280, "Why We Need a Code of Professional Ethics," Aug. 25, 1999, http://www.nteu280.org/issues/nteu-20%professional %20Ethics.htm (accessed June 14, 2001).

35. Ibid.

36. On the "view from nowhere," see Haraway, "Situated Knowledges."

37. For a detailed analysis of how this worked at the EPA in the case of carpet, see the five-part series by the activist Cindy Duehring, beginning with "Carpet."

38. For two union members' versions of these events, see Hirzy and Morison, "Carpet/4-Psheylcyclohexene Toxicity."

39. Anderson Laboratories, "Carpet Offgassing." Anderson Labs used a standard experimental protocol called ASTM-E981. It involved restraining mice in an environmental chamber and blowing hot air over an item, in this case carpet, and onto the mice for discrete length of time. The mice were then assessed for changes in respiratory and pulmonary function through the protocol's established measure. Unlike the experimental design that connected lead to lead poisoning, ASTM-E981 could test objects and the variety of chemicals they omitted, and not just one specific chemical. This

experiment's findings were eventually published in Rosalind Anderson, "Toxic Emissions."

40. Victor J. Kimm, acting assistant administrator for prevention, pesticides, and toxic substances, U.S. EPA, testimony before the House Committee on Government Operations, Subcommittee on Environment, Energy, and Natural Resources, *Potential Risks of Carpet and Carpeting Materials*, 103rd Congress, 1st sess., June 11, 1993. See also the report on experiments at DuPont and Monsanto, Stadler et al., "Evaluation."

41. In courtroom litigation about toxic effects alleged to be caused by carpet, the defense had Anderson's expert testimony stricken from evidence based on a 1993 Supreme Court ruling, *Daubert v. Merrell Dow Pharmaceuticals*, which had established a new set of standards for judging scientific evidence, including peer review and independent replication of findings. *Sandra Ruffin; Catherin Ruffin v. Shaw Industries, Incorporated; Sherwin-Williams Company*, 94–1882 (4th Cir. Ct. of Appeals, 1998).

42. See, e.g., Harding, "Feminist Empiricism"; Harstock, "Comment"; and Lukács, "Reification."

43. Huginnie, "Containment."

44. Beck, *Risk Society*.

45. *White Noise* was published at the same time as the Bhopal chemical disaster occurred, so that coverage of Bhopal in the mainstream press and reviews of the novel were occurring simultaneously.

46. This description of Waterside Mall is compiled from my own observations during a visit in 1996, press coverage of the indoor pollution episode, the Indoor Air Quality and Work Environment Survey, and, most important, the approximately twelve hundred essays EPA employees wrote on the back of this survey, administered in Feb. 1989. The essay responses were compiled in an unpublished manuscript: Wallace, "Preliminary Analysis."

47. Wallace, "Preliminary Analysis," 6–9.

48. These symptoms were recorded in the health survey handed out by Local 2050 at the May 25, 1988, protest. NFFE Papers, NFFE office, U.S. Environmental Protection Agency National Headquarters, Washington, D.C.

49. This meeting and quote was reported in the *Washington Times*, beginning what was to become a torrent of articles in Washington, D.C., newspapers; Vukelich, "Employees." The quote was also corroborated in interviews I conducted with Local 2050 leaders in 1996. The air monitoring was eventually written up in Singhvi, Turpin, and Burchette, "Final Summary Report."

50. Wallace, *Total Exposure*.

51. Wallace, interview with author, Washington, D.C., April 30, 1996.

52. U.S. EPA, *Indoor Air Quality*.

53. *Bahura v. S.E.W. Investors et al.*, No. 90CA10594 (D.C. S. Ct. 1995). The jury came to their conclusion with the help of expert witness Abba Terr, who testifies around the country that multiple chemical sensitivity is a psychosomatic illness.

54. Carol Browner, administrator of the U.S. EPA, testimony before the House Committee on Science, *Intolerance at EPA: Harming People, Harming Science?*, 106th Congress, 2nd sess., Oct. 4, 2000.

55. U.S. Senate Banking Committee, "Senator Gramm's Letter."

56. *Coleman-Adebayo v. Carol Browner, U.S. Environmental Protection Agency*, No. 1.98cv 1939 (U.S. Dist. Ct., Washington, D.C., Aug. 18, 2000).

57. Leroy W. Warren Jr., chairman of the NAACP Federal Sector Task Force, testimony before the House Committee on Science, *Intolerance at EPA: Harming People, Harming Science?* 106th Congress, 2nd sess., Oct. 4, 2000.

58. Jack White, "How the EPA."

59. Header of the EPAVRD Web site, http://www.epavard.org (accessed April 16, 2001).

60. Notification and Federal Employee Anti-discrimination and Retaliation Act of 2001 bill, H.R. 169, Introduction to the House, 106th Congress, 2d sess., *Congressional Record*, Jan. 3, 2001.

6. Building Ecologies and Tobacco

1. On personal clouds, see the epilogue and Wallace, "TEAM Studies."

2. On the history of ecology and ecosystems ecology, see Hagen, *Entangled Bank*; McIntosh, *Background of Ecology*; and Mitman, *State of Nature*.

3. Hagen, *Entangled Bank*, 127.

4. Heims, *Constructing a Social Science*.

5. Taylor, "Technocratic Optimism."

6. H. T. Odum, "Ecological Potential"; Taylor, "Technocratic Optimism."

7. Howard Odum, *Environment*, 1.

8. Eugene Odum, *Ecology*, 4.

9. Eugene Odum, *Fundamentals of Ecology*, 3.

10. E. P. Odum, quoted in McIntosh, *Background of Ecology*, 228, and Eugene Odum, *Ecology*, v.

11. Eugene Odum, *Ecology*, 216.

12. Howard Odum, *Environment*, 1.

13. Ibid., 140.

14. Hagen, *Entangled Bank*, 139; Taylor, "Technocratic Optimism."

15. The founding document in organizational ecology is Freeman and Hannan, "Population Ecology." See also Carroll, *Ecological Models*; and Hannan and Freeman, *Organization Ecology*.

16. Moore, *Death of Competition.*

17. James Martin, *Cybercorp,* 3.

18. Ibid.

19. From book jacket description; Hasenyager, *Managing.*

20. Drucker, *Ecological Vision.*

21. Becker and Steele, *Workplace by Design.* See also Steele, *Making and Managing.*

22. Bauer, *Second-Order Consequences.*

23. Gunn and Burroughs, "Work Spaces That Work," 20.

24. The Steelcase Worklife New York opened in 1997; http://www.steel case.com/viewnew/nwlnyfs.html (accessed Nov. 23, 1997). See also Peter-sen, "Metaphor of a Corporate Display."

25. On the relationship between buildings and bodies, see Collins, *Changing Ideals*; Diller and Scofidio, *Flesh*; Pouchelle, *Body and Surgery*; Sennet, *Flesh and Stone*; and Stafford, *Body Criticism.*

26. Hal Levin, "Healthy Buildings."

27. Fraser et al., "Legionnaires' Disease"; O'Mahoney et al., "Legion-naires' Disease."

28. Arnow et al., "Early Detection"; Banaszak, Thiede, and Fink, "Hyper-sensitivity Pneumonitis"; Edwards, Griffiths, and Mullins, "Protozoa"; Fin-negan and Pickering, "Review: Building Related Illness"; Garnier et al., "Humidifier Lung"; Hodges, Fink, and Schlueter, "Hypersensitivity Pneu-monitis"; Kohler, "Medical Reform"; Weiss and Solemanyi, "Hypersen-sitivity Lung Disease."

29. Hoy, *Chasing Dirt*; Tomes, *Gospel of Germs.*

30. Haraway, "Biopolitics"; Emily Martin, *Flexible Bodies.*

31. See, e.g., William Clark, *At War Within*; Dwyer, *Body at War*; Jaret, "Our Immune System"; and Nilsson, *Body Victorious.*

32. Odatus, *Immune System for Buildings,* http://www.odatus.com (ac-cessed Dec. 10, 1997).

33. http://www.honeywell.com (accessed Dec. 10, 1997).

34. Hal Levin, "Building Ecology."

35. Levin and Teichman, "Indoor Air Quality," 57.

36. Whorton et al., "Investigation and Work-Up," 147.

37. Hicks, "Tight Building Syndrome," 54.

38. Hearing on the Indoor Air Quality Act of 1988, House Committee on Sci-ence, Space, and Technology, Subcommittee on Natural Resources, Agricul-ture Research, and Environment, 100th Congress, 2nd sess., Sept. 28, 1988. No. 152 (Washington, D.C., U.S. Government Printing Office), 120–50.

39. Vischer, "Environmental Quality," 123.

40. World Health Organization, "Indoor Air Pollutants."

41. Ventilation engineers at ASHRAE had long ago learned that the quality

of the environment could only be assessed through the human body. If at all possible, however, the human body was to be assessed by physiological instruments, and only when these failed by subjective judgments. Yet even in the earliest environmental chamber experiments, discussed in chap. 1, the quality of the environment was ultimately determined, not by the instruments that rationally measured variables but by the votes of experimental subjects, who in turn were guided by their noses. Even the ASHRAE building codes produced by these experiments and inscribed in the construction of office buildings were policed by the use of the human nose. It still remains established protocol to judge a building's air quality by a panel of untrained noses: "In the absence of objective means to assess the acceptability of such contaminants, the judgment of acceptability must necessarily derive from the subjective evaluation of impartial observers. The air can be considered acceptably free of annoying contaminants if 80% of a panel of at least 20 untrained observers deems the air to be not objectionable under representative conditions of use and occupation" ("Ventilation for Acceptable Indoor Air Quality," ASHRAE Standard, 62–1989). Absorbing this ASHRAE measure, the threshold at which a building was typically declared "sick" became the moment when over 20% of its occupants reported symptoms. Thus, the measure that determined a "sick building" was the proportion of workers that experienced symptoms, not the kinds of symptoms or their cause. Questionnaires, however, differ from the ASHRAE measure in that they rely on building occupants who spend their whole day indoors, not impartial, visiting observers who "should render a judgment of acceptability within 15 seconds" (ASHRAE Standard, 62–1989).

42. See, e.g., Kangmin Zhu, "Letter to the Editor."

43. Jameson, *Postmodernism*, xii.

44. Stolwijk (1991), "Sick-Building Syndrome," 100.

45. Odatus, *Immune System for Buildings*, http://www.odatus.com (accessed Dec. 10, 1997).

46. Myron Levin, "Who's Behind the Building Doctor?"; Mintz, "Smoke Screen."

47. Using its own building investigations as the data, HBI often cited its estimate that tobacco smoke played a role in 3% of SBS cases. However, this obscures incidents when tobacco smoke might have been named as an irritant unassociated with any larger SBS episode.

48. The CIAR was disbanded in 1998 as part of the Master Settlement Agreement.

49. On the sponsorship of Robertson, see Mintz, "Smoke Screen." For a list of buildings the firm investigated, see References, Healthy Buildings International, Web site, http://www.hbiamerica.com/references/index.htm (accessed Nov. 19, 2003).

50. Myron Levin, "Who's Behind the Building Doctor?"; Mintz, "Smoke Screen."

51. Healthy Buildings International, "Sick Building Syndrome Causes and Cures," 1991. Legacy Tobacco Documents Library, Philip Morris Collection, Bates No. 2022889309–9324, http://legacy.library.ucsf.edu/tid/hpc78e00 (accessed Nov. 27, 2003).

52. "Business Council on Indoor Air: A Multi-industry Response," 6.

53. Gray Robertson, Healthy Buildings International, *Sick Building Syndrome—Facts and Fallacies*, Oct. 23, 1991, Legacy Tobacco Documents Library, R. J. Reynolds, Bates No. 509915547–5568, http://legacy.library.ucsf.edu/tid/qbr63d00. Recent Advances in Tobacco Science, v. 17. Topics of Current Scientific Interest in Tobacco Research, Proceedings of a Symposium Presented at the Forty-Fifth Meeting of the Tobacco Chemists' Research Conference (accessed Nov. 27, 2003): 151–52.

54. Healthy Buildings International, "HBI Experience."

55. HBI's relationship with the tobacco industry was revealed in 1992 when a fired employee turned whistle-blower. By 1998 the Master Settlement Agreement, a settlement between the U.S. state attorneys general and major tobacco companies, along with the Tobacco Institute, mandated that the industry release digital snapshots of millions of pages of internal documents, which have since demonstrated the industry's support of indoor air quality research and investigators, establishing ties not only with Robertson but a host of other indoor air quality specialists.

56. U.S. Environmental Protection Agency, "Indoor Air Facts." Much of the credit for the successful publication of this pamphlet is due to James Repace, a senior EPA scientist, whistle-blower, and active NFFE union member, who widely published his rebuttals to the tobacco industry. On the EPA's building assessment approach, see U.S. Environmental Protection Agency and National Institute of Occupational Safety and Health, "Building Air Quality."

57. Healthy Buildings International, "About Us," http://www.hbiamerica.com/aboutus/index.htm (accessed Nov. 11, 2003).

58. Ibid.

59. Gray Robertson, "Sick Building Syndrome," Nov. 18, 1987, Legacy Tobacco Documents Library, Philip Morris Collection, Bates No. 2061692010-2012, http://legacy.library.ucsf.edu/tid/pjf49e00 (accessed Nov. 27, 2003).

60. See, e.g., the role of tobacco industry representatives within ASHRAE; Glantz and Bialous, "ASHRAE Standard 62."

61. Business Council on Indoor Air, "Indoor Air Quality: A Public Health Issue in the 1990s; How Will It Affect Your Company?," undated brochure, received on April 11, 1996, and "Building Systems Approach."

62. "Labor Indoor Air Quality Presentations and Events," Jan. 1990, Legacy

Tobacco Documents Library, Tobacco Institute, Bates No. TI02120328-0338, http://legacy.library.ucsf.edu/tid/wht30c00 (accessed Nov. 23, 2003).

63. "Investigating the 'Sick Building Syndrome': ETS in Context," statement of Gray Robertson, president, ACVA Atlantic, Inc., before the National Academy of Sciences Concerning the Contribution of Environmental Tobacco Smoke to Indoor Air Pollution, Jan. 14, 1986, Legacy Tobacco Documents Library, Philip Morris Collection, Bates No. 2021005103-5125, http://legacy.library.ucsf.edu/tid/epj34e00 (accessed Nov. 27, 2003), 7.

64. U.S. Environmental Protection Agency and National Institute of Occupational Safety and Health, "Building Air Quality," x.

65. Robertson, "Investigating the 'Sick Building Syndrome,'" 21.

7. A Body in a Safe Space

1. The messy controversy around environmental illness is complicated by both the multiplicity of names used and the lack of a single definition. However, one offered by Mark Cullen has proved useful and influential: "Multiple chemical sensitivities (MCS) is an acquired disorder characterized by recurrent symptoms, referable to multiple organ systems, occurring in response to demonstrable exposure to many chemical unrelated compounds at doses far below those established in the general population to cause harmful effects. No single widely accepted physiological function can be shown to correlate with symptoms"; Cullen, *Workers*, 657.

2. Though individual physicians may be sympathetic to MCS, the diagnosis and the allied field of clinical ecology were overwhelmingly criticized by medical associations in a series of position papers; American Academy of Allergy and Immunology, "Position Statements"; American College of Physicians, "Position Paper"; American Medical Association, "Council Report"; American Psychiatric Association, *Diagnostic and Statistical Manual*; California Medical Association, "Clinical Ecology."

3. American Psychiatric Association, *Diagnostic and Statistical Manual*, 445. For examples of works that substitute a psychosomatic diagnosis for MCS, see Gori, "Role of Objective Science"; Gothe, Odont, and Nilsson, "Environmental Somatization Syndrome"; Gots, *Toxic Risks*; Simon, Katon, and Sparks, "Allergic to Life"; Staudenmayer and Selner, "Failure to Assess Psychopathology"; and Terr, "Environmental Illness."

4. A Denver allergist and psychiatrist team undertook a double-blind study with an environmental chamber to try to reproduce the symptoms that twenty MCS sufferers claimed to suffer from. They failed; Staudenmayer, Selner, and Buhr, "Double-Blind Provacation." This study was an important part of the argument against the validity of MCS considered by medical

associations. The two doctors rediagnosed these patients as having psychiatric problems needing therapy. As a result, they set up a clinic that attached an allergy practice to a psychiatric practice.

5. American Psychiatric Association, *Diagnostic and Statistical Manual*, 445.

6. Testimony by clinical ecologists concerning multiple chemical sensitivity was deemed inadmissible through a ruling in the 1997 federal case *Daubert v. Merrell Dow Pharmaceuticals*. The ruling hinged on the lack of an objective testing method for MCS and the rejection of the allied field of clinical ecology by the American Medical Association and the American College of Physicians. On the role of medical testimony in the court, see Bertin and Henifin, "Science, Law"; Brickman, Jasanoff, and Ilgen, *Controlling Chemicals*; Jasanoff, "Science, Politics"; and Jasanoff, *Science at the Bar*.

7. Butler, *Bodies That Matter*, 3. On abjection, also see Kristeva, *Powers of Horror*.

8. This appellation is mobilized by Ronald Gots, the most outspoken of the MCS debunkers.

9. Schlesinger, "'Letter,'" 1. Hilde Schlesinger was president of the Environmental Health Network, a San Francisco–area organization for the environmentally sensitive.

10. E-mail, Immune list (March 8, 1996).

11. E-mail, MCS-CI list (Feb. 5, 1998).

12. Cynthia Wilson, "Disposable Cogs." Wilson is a vocal advocate within the MCS movement. Located in Montana, she is editor of one of its most important newsletters, *Our Toxic Times*.

13. *New Reactor* 5, no. 3 (May–Oct. 1995), 9.

14. This is the title of a book written by a nurse with MCS; Witteberg, *Rebellious Body*.

15. This name comes from a very moving photographic exhibit of people living with MCS by Rhonda Zwillinger, who herself suffers with MCS; Zwillinger, *Dispossessed*.

16. Gots, "Medical Hypothesis"; Shorter, *Paralysis to Fatigue*; Shorter, *Mind into the Body*; Shorter, "Borderland"; Showalter, *Hystories*.

17. Patient perspective histories have tended to assume that we can recover the experience of the sick person and thereby give that experience a voice that has been unheard or unspoken. By making visible and granting authority to "experience," such scholarship attempts to empower victims, yet often at the expense of accepting identities as natural categories. Thus, categories like *woman* and *sickness* are assumed to be prior to history, even if historical circumstances grant them meaning. In this way, experience becomes an origin of explanation and a type of uncontested knowledge, leaving unquestioned the very terms and structures that constituted the patient,

woman, or worker as invisible or outside. For a more detailed account of the historicity of experience, see chap. 3.

18. See, e.g., Gibson, "Environmental Illness."

19. Dumit, "Invisible Emerging Illnesses"; Mike Fortun, "Defining Disease"; Kroll-Smith and Floyd, *Bodies in Protest*; Naismith, "Tales from the Crypt."

20. Eisenberg et al., "Unconventional Medicine."

21. Deleuze described nomadization as travel in which one does not migrate from point *A* to point *B*, but rather moves in order to stay in the same place by freeing oneself from the grids that map us; Deleuze, "Pensée nomade," 176.

22. My description of cellular "new social movements" is taken from the works of the sociologist Alberto Melucci, *Nomads of the Present* and *Challenging Code*. For an essay that uses Melucci to describe alternative health, see Schneirov and Geczik, "Diagnosis."

23. Epstein, *Impure Science*.

24. Murphy, "Hearing Gulf War Syndrome."

25. The phrase "elsewhere within here" comes from Trinh Minh-Ha, *Woman, Native, Other*. Partially building on Trinh, Donna Haraway describes the "elsewhere" as an excursion for theorizing between nature and artifactualism "to produce a patterned vision of how to move and what to fear in the topography of an impossible but all-too-real present, in order to find an absent, but perhaps possible, other present"; Haraway, "Promises of Monsters," 295.

26. This is paraphrased from "you intervene even as you inhabit those structures"; Spivak, *Post-colonial Critic*, 72.

27. Foucault, "Technologies of the Self," 18.

28. "What can I do, what power can I claim and what resistances may I encounter? What can I be, with what folds can I surround myself or how can I produce myself as a subject? On these three questions, the 'I' does not designate a universal but a set of particular positions occupied with a One speaks, One sees, One confronts, One lives"; Deleuze, *Foucault*, 114–15. For an excellent, but difficult, reading of Foucault's theory of subjectivity and technologies of the self, see the chapter "Foldings, or the Inside of Thought (Subjectivation)," 94–123.

29. For a feminist therapy perspective discussion of MCS as invisible disability, see Gibson, "Environmental Illness."

30. Chavkin, *Double Exposure*. It is important to note here that while there is a gendering of chemical exposure through housework, this does not apply to commercial built environments, where chemical exposures around cleaning products are more likely racialized. The maintenance of work spaces tended to be segregated by race or immigration status. Further, upper-mid-

dle-class white women employed women of color to clean their homes. Glenn, "Servitude to Service Work." This raises the question, *Why are these workers not more involved in the MCS movement?* I would suggest that there is a politics at work here by which the identity of "victim" is not as available or viable for men and women of color, particularly if they are not granted citizenship status, as it is for relatively privileged white women, particularly from the middle class, who are citizens and eligible to appeal to state protection. This disparity in the use of "victim" identities has been a significant problematic within feminist scholarship. White feminists have been criticized as overly eager to recognize their victim status while ignoring their role in perpetuating racism, colonialism, and other inequalities. U.S. feminists of color have often taken an alternative strategy of constituting nonvictim identities around strength and survival; Wendy Brown, *States of Injury*; Hull, Bell, and Smith, *All the Women Are White*; Mohanty, "Feminist Encounters."

31. This history is largely culled from Dickey, *Clinical Ecology*; and Randolph, "Allergy and Clinical Ecology."

32. Dickey, *Clinical Ecology*, 743. It is ironic that clinical ecologists used the term *man* in their writings when most of their patients were women and children.

33. Eugene Odum, "Emergence of Ecology," 1289. This article is quoted at length in Randolph, *Environmental Medicine*, 203–4.

34. Rea et al., "Confirmation."

35. Gots, "Medical Hypothesis"; Gots, "Multiple Chemical Sensitivities"; Terr, "Environmental Illness"; Terr, "'Multiple Chemical Sensitivities.'" A majority of ESRI's board members represent industries, such as Amway, Bayer, Colgate-Palmolive, DowElanco, the Chemical Specialty Manufacturers Association, the Cosmetic, Toiletry, and Fragrance Association, and Proctor and Gamble.

36. It was later renamed the International Center for Toxicology and Medicine.

37. After *Daubert v. Merrell Dow Pharmaceuticals Inc.*, clinical ecologists were no longer allowed to give expert testimony or diagnose environmental illness in court cases (see n. 6 in this chapter).

38. Many of the new practitioners in clinical ecology had themselves suffered from MCS or environmental sensitivities; Rea et al., "Chemical Sensitivity."

39. Rea et al., "Considerations," 171.

40. Kroll-Smith and Floyd, *Bodies in Protest*.

41. Disability benefits from Social Security are determined by ability to function, rather than by cause and effect. To obtain disability benefits as a sufferer of MCS, one often must pursue the case in court. (Here we are back in court again.) The difficulties involved in qualifying for disability benefits

with a diagnosis of MCS lead many to resort to filing a claim of mental disability. This decision is very difficult to make. Some MCSers feel that filing under mental disability is "selling out." Others argue that mental disability is the result, not the cause, of MCS, and, moreover, that one should not reinforce the stigmatization of the mentally ill. Workplace accommodation is covered by the Americans with Disabilities Act, under which MCS is technically included. However, accommodation for MCSers, be it by employers or public services, has been resisted fiercely in the courts.

42. On the history of domestic space as gendered, see Hayden, *Grand Domestic Revolution*; and Wright, *Building the Dream*.

43. On the history of housework and cleanliness, see Ruth Schwartz Cowan, *More Work*; Hoy, *Chasing Dirt*; and Tomes, *Gospel of Germs*.

44. These specialty products are usually sold by small home businesses run by MCSers themselves.

45. See, e.g., Duehring and Wilson, *Human Consequences*; Lawson, *Staying Well*; Cynthia Wilson, *Chemical Exposure*; and Witteberg, *Rebellious Body*.

46. While MCSers are stereotyped as upper-middle-class housewives, such as those portrayed in the Todd Haynes movie *Safe* (1993), many are working women, part of the "pink-collar" working class employed in information or service jobs. With the advent of illness, many MCSers either quit or loose their jobs and join the ranks of the functionally unemployable.

47. Ad in the *New Reactor* (Jan.–Feb. 1996).

48. Ad in *Our Toxic Times* (Dec. 1996).

49. Ad in *Our Toxic Times* (July 1996).

50. In Louisville, Ky., for example, the local MCS support group planned, but did not succeed in building, a safe village called Norton Commons.

51. "Word from God," May 17, 1996, quoted on the Alpha Omega Christian Communities for the Chemically Injured Web site; http://www.intx .net/aoccci (accessed March 18, 1998).

52. Beck, *Risk Society*.

53. Garreau, *Edge City*.

54. Watney, *Policing Desire*.

55. An important part of my research into MCS has taken place on the Internet. For example, I subscribed to the Immune list from 1993 to 1998.

56. Formal description of purpose of the MCS-Immune-Neuro list (Jan. 6, 1997).

57. E-mail, Immune list (Feb. 18, 1996).

58. Haraway, "Biopolitics."

59. The anthropologist Emily Martin, in her book *Flexible Bodies*, which follows immune systems from science to popular media to popular culture, argues that they are particularly postmodern objects tightly linked to late-capitalist economies of flexible accumulation.

60. E.g., Irun Cohen, "Self, World."

61. Rogers, *Tired or Toxic?*

62. E-mail, Immune list (Feb. 19, 1996).

63. E-mail, MCS-Immune-Neuro list (Nov. 8, 1997).

64. Quoted from the Alpha Omega Christian Communities for the Chemically Injured Web site; http://www.intx.net/aoccci (accessed March 18, 1998).

65. The archive of postings from the Immune list has a special section collecting all posts that deal with emotions, mind-body, and child abuse; http://www.best.com/~immune/emotionrefs.html. This argument about brain chemistry is also used by those who want to classify MCS as a psychosomatic illness, contending that the brain scans MCSers use to objectify their illness only prove that emotions have biological effects on the body.

66. It is important to note that the MCS movement, despite the unequal distribution of chemical exposures by race and economic status, is predominantly, though not absolutely, composed of white women. One cultural explanation for this racialization of MCS may be that white women are more likely to pursue medicalization and medical diagnosis than women of color. Though whiteness is not explicitly a part of the MCS identity, "race" seems to be doing cultural work, shaping who participates in the movement.

67. On these performances in relation to eating disorders, see Bordo, *Unbearable Weight.*

68. "Our Stolen Future."

69. This phrase is partially a citation of Deleuze and Guattari's injunction to build yourself a "body without organs." I believe an important, though often underplayed, aspect of this injunction is the warning to proceed with caution; Deleuze and Guattari, *Thousand Plateaus.*

70. E-mail, Immune list (May 1994).

71. E-mail, MCS-Immune-Neuro list (Sept. 17, 1997).

72. Ibid.

73. Ibid.

74. This aspect of the MCS movement is very disturbing to the debunkers of MCS, such as Ronald Gots, who wrote, "The 1960s brought empowerment of the public, holistic medicine, and a decline generally in public esteem of science and medicine. . . . The public became actively participatory, with the help of sympathetic physicians, in defining health issues including causes of disease. Thus, each individual became a personal laboratory, 'understanding' his or her own body, 'knowing' how various factors or substances influenced it. In effect, the science of medicine gave way to these newly encouraged personal testimonials and anecdotal reports, and physicians became more mere chroniclers of these popular anecdotes than students of disease causation. The net effect of this 'enlightenment' on the

science of medicine has been as negative as the 'discovery' of autointoxication. Gross misperceptions existed then about the causes of disease and they
continue to exist today"; Gots, *Toxic Risks*. In response to Gots, some MCSers
have informally formed a "Get Gots Gang," which researches Gots's activities and background and then publicizes them at events. Albert Donnay
of MCS Referral and Resources, an advocacy and information service in the
Baltimore area, is a central actor in this type of activism. Gots and MCS R and
R are direct antagonists and have even debated each other on the radio
(*Sunday Rounds*, NPR, Baltimore, Nov. 11, 1995). Donnay was most effective
in his "Get Gots" efforts when he publicized Gots's involvement in an international MCS workshop, which convened in Berlin (Feb. 21–25, 1995) under
the auspices of the World Health Organization (WHO), the United Nations
Environmental Program, and the International Labor Organization (ILO).
The workshop concluded that "MCS cannot be regarded as a clinically defined disease." It advocated using the term *ideopathic environmental intolerance* (IEI), which removes the word "chemical" as found in MCS. Donnay
publicized that the workshop was actually sponsored by the industry-boost-
ing International Program on Chemical Safety (IPCS) and that the members
of the workshop had close ties to industry. A letter signed by over fifty
environmental health experts was sent to the IPCS, the UN, the ILO, and
WHO protesting the conclusions of the workshop; Donnay, "MCS or IEI?";
John Wilson, "Gots Misrepresents Workshop."

75. E-mail, Immune list (Sept. 1994).

76. Ibid.

Epilogue

1. Wallace, *Total Exposure*.

2. In fact, such dogs were programmed in the Feral Robotic Dog project of
Natalie Jeremijenko, where teenagers from the Bronx and Orlando hacked
store-bought robotic dogs to include environmental sensors; http://xdesign
.eng.yale.edu/feralrobots/ (accessed Dec. 8, 2003).

3. In fact, the CDC has just begun to do something similar; U.S. Centers
for Disease Control and Prevention, *Second National Report*.

4. See, e.g., Welshons et al., "Large Effects."

5. See, e.g., Rajapakse, Silva, and Kortenkamp, "Combining Xenoestrogens."

Ackerknecht, Erwin. "Anticontagionism between 1821 and 1867." *Bulletin of the History of Medicine* 22 (1948): 562–93.

Ackerman, Marsha E. *Cool Comfort: America's Romance with Air-Conditioning.* Washington, D.C.: Smithsonian Institute Press, 2002.

Albert, Margie. "Something New in the Women's Movement." *New York Times,* Dec. 12, 1973.

Allan, Barbara. *Uneasy Alchemy: Citizens and Experts in Louisiana's Chemical Corridor Disputes.* Cambridge: MIT Press, 2003.

Althusser, Louis. "Ideology and Ideological State Apparatuses." In *Lenin and Philosophy,* 127–86. New York: Monthly Review Press, 1977.

American Academy of Allergy and Immunology. "Position Statements: Clinical Ecology." *Journal of Allergy and Clinical Immunology* 78 (Aug. 1986): 269–71.

American College of Physicians. "Position Paper: Clinical Ecology." *Annals of Internal Medicine* 111, no. 2 (1989): 168–78.

American Medical Association. "Council Report: Clinical Ecology." *JAMA* 268, no. 24 (1992): 3465–67.

American Psychiatric Association. *Diagnostic and Statistical Manual of Mental Disorders.* 4th ed. Washington, D.C.: American Psychiatric Association, 1994.

Anderson, Rosalind. "Toxic Emissions from Carpets." *Journal of Nutritional and Environmental Medicine* 5 (1995): 375–86.

Anderson, Warwick. "The Trespass Speaks: White Masculinity and Colonial Breakdown." *American Historical Review* 102, no. 5 (1997): 1343–70.

Anderson Laboratories. "Carpet Offgassing and Lethal Effects on Mice." Press release, Aug. 18, 1992.

Arnow, Paul, et al. "Early Detection of Hypersensitivity Pneumonitis in Office Workers." *American Journal of Medicine* 64, no. 2 (1978): 236–41.

Aron, Cindy Sondik. *Ladies and Gentlemen of the Civil Service: Middle Class Workers in Victorian America.* New York: Oxford University Press, 1987.

ASHVE Research Technical Advisory Committee on Physiological Reactions. "Recent Advances in Physiological Knowledge and Their Bearing on Ventilation Practice." *Transactions* 45 (1939): 111–21.

Atkinson, J. "Manpower Strategies for Flexible Organizations." *Personnel Management*, Aug. 1984.

Bale, Anthony. " 'Hope in Another Direction': Compensation for Work-Related Illness among Women, 1900–1960, Part I." *Women and Health* 14 (1989): 81–102.

——. " 'Hope in Another Direction': Compensation for Work-Related Illness among Women, 1900–1960, Part II." *Women and Health* 15 (1989): 99–115.

Banaszak, E. F., W. H. Thiede, and J. N. Fink. "Hypersensitivity Pneumonitis Due to Contamination of an Air Conditioner." *New England Journal of Medicine* 283 (1970): 271–76.

Banham, Reyner. *Theory and Design in the First Machine Age*. 2nd. ed. New York: Praeger, 1967.

——. *The Architecture of the Well-Tempered Environment*. Chicago: University of Chicago Press, 1969.

Banning, Margaret. "Workplace Chemicals Put the Emphasis on Occupational Health." *Monitor*, May 1984, 16–17.

Banta, Martha. *Taylored Lives: Narrative Productions in the Age of Taylor, Veblen, and Ford*. Chicago: University of Chicago Press, 1993.

Barker, Jane, and Hazel Downing. "Word Processing and the Transformation of Patriarchal Relations of Control in the Office." In *The Social Shaping of Technology: How the Refrigerator Got Its Hum*, edited by Donald MacKenzie and Judy Wajcman, 147–64. Milton Keynes, U.K.: Open University Press, 1985.

Barnes, Deborah, and Lisa Biro. "Industry-Funded Research in Conflict of Interest: An Analysis of Research Sponsored by the Tobacco Industry through the Center for Indoor Air Research." *Journal of Health Politics, Policy and Law* 21, no. 3: 515.

Bates, E. P. "President's Remarks." *ASHVE Transactions* 1 (1895).

Bauer, Raymond. *Second-Order Consequences: A Methodological Essay on the Impact of Technology*. Cambridge: MIT Press, 1969.

Bauer, Russel, Kevin Greve, et al. "The Role of Psychological Factors in the Report of Building-Related Symptoms in Sick Building Syndrome." *Journal of Consulting and Clinical Psychology* 60, no. 2 (1992): 213–19.

Bay, Mia. " 'The World Was Thinking Wrong about Race': *The Philadelphia Negro* and Nineteenth-Century Science." In *W. E. B. DuBois, Race, and the City: "The Philadelphia Negro" and Its Legacy*, edited by Michael Katz and Thomas Sugrue, 41–60. Philadelphia: University of Pennsylvania Press, 1998.

Bayer, Ronald, ed. *The Health and Safety of Workers: Case Studies in the Politics of Professional Responsibility*. New York: Oxford University Press, 1988.

Beck, Ulrich. "From Industrial Society to the Risk Society: Questions of

Survival, Social Structure and Ecological Enlightenment." In *Cultural Theory and Cultural Change*, edited by Mike Featherstone, 97–123. London: Sage, 1992.

———. *Risk Society: Towards a New Modernity*. Translated by Mark Ritter. London: Sage, 1992.

Becker, Franklin, and Fritz Steele. *Workplace by Design: Mapping the High-Performance Workscape*. San Francisco: Jossey-Bass, 1995.

Bell, Deborah. "Unionized Women in State and Local Government." In *Women, Work and Protest*, edited by Ruth Milkman, 280–99. Boston: Routledge and Keegan Paul, 1985.

Bellamy, Elizabeth, and Artemis Leontis. "A Genealogy of Experience: From Epistemology to Politics." *Yale Journal of Criticism* 6, no. 1 (1993): 163–84.

Bennett, Amanda. *The Death of Organization Man*. New York: William Morrow, 1990.

Bensaude-Vincent, Bernadette, and Isabelle Stengers. *A History of Chemistry*. Translated by Deborah van Dam. Cambridge: Harvard University Press, 1997.

Berman, Daniel. "Why Work Kills: A Brief History of Occupational Safety and Health in the United States." *International Journal of Health Services* 7 (1977): 63–87.

Bertin, Joan, and Mary Henifin. "Science, Law and the Search for Truth in the Courtroom: Lessons from *Daubert v. Merrell Dow*." *Journal of Law, Medicine, and Ethics* 22, no. 1 (1995): 6–20.

Biggs, Lindy. *The Rational Factory*. Baltimore: Johns Hopkins University Press, 1996.

Blum, Elizabeth. "Pink and Green: A Comparative Study of Black Activism in the Twentieth Century." PhD diss., University of Houston, 2000.

Boden, Leslie. "Problems in Occupational Disease Compensation." In *Current Issues in Workers' Compensation*, edited by James Chelius, 313–25. Kalamazoo, Mich.: W. E. Upjohn Institute for Employment Research, 1986.

Borchert, James. *Alley Life in Washington: Family, Community, Religion and Folklife in the City, 1850–1970*. Urbana: University of Illinois Press, 1980.

Bordo, Susan. *Unbearable Weight: Feminism, Western Culture, and the Body*. Berkeley: University of California Press, 1993.

Botsch, Robert. *Organizing the Breathless: Cotton Dust, Southern Politics and the Brown Lung Association*. Lexington: University Press of Kentucky, 1993.

Boxer, Peter. "Occupational Mass Psychogenic Illness." *Journal of Occupational Medicine* 27, no. 12 (1985): 867–72.

Branchaw, Bernadine, et al. *Office Procedures for the Professional Secretary*. Chicago: Science Research Associates Inc., 1984.

Braverman, Harry. *Labor and Monopoly Capital: The Degradation of Work in the Twentieth Century*. New York: Monthly Review Press, 1974.

Brickman, Ronald, Sheila Jasanoff, and Thomas Ilgen. *Controlling Chemicals: The Politics of Regulation in Europe and the United States*. Ithaca, N.Y.: Cornell University Press, 1985.

Briskin, Linda, and Patricia McDermott, eds. *Women Challenging Unions: Feminism, Democracy, and Militancy*. Toronto: University of Toronto Press, 1993.

Brock, William. *The Norton History of Chemistry*. Edited by Roy Porter. Norton History of Science. New York: W. W. Norton and Company, 1992.

Brown, Phil. "Popular Epidemiology: Community Response to Toxic Waste-Induced Disease in Woburn, Massachusetts." *Science, Technology, and Human Values* 12 (1987): 78–85.

Brown, Phil, and Faith Ferguson. " 'Making a Big Stink': Women's Work, Women's Relationships and Toxic Waste Activism." *Gender and Society* 9, no. 2 (1995): 145–72.

Brown, Phil, and Edwin J. Mikkelsen. *No Safe Place: Toxic Waste, Leukemia, and Community Action*. Berkeley: University of California Press, 1990.

Brown, Wendy. *States of Injury: Power and Freedom in Late Modernity*. Princeton, N.J: Princeton University Press, 1995.

Bryant, Bunyan, and Paul Mohai. "Environmental Injustice: Weighing Race and Class as Factors in the Distribution of Environmental Hazards." *University of Colorado Law Review* 63, no. 4 (1992): 921–32.

Bullard, Robert. "Environmental Justice for All." In *Unequal Protection: Environmental Justice and Communities of Color*, edited by Robert Bullard, 3–22. San Francisco: Sierra Club Books, 1994.

———, ed. *Confronting Environmental Racism: Voices from the Grassroots*. Cambridge, Mass.: South End, 1993.

Bulmer, Martin. "The Decline of the Social Survey Movement and the Rise of American Empirical Sociology." In *The Social Survey in Historical Perspective, 1880–1940*, edited by Martin Bulmer, Kevin Bales, and Kathryn Kish Sklar, 291–315. Cambridge: Cambridge University Press, 1991.

———. "W. E. B. Du Bois as a Social Investigatory: *The Philadelphia Negro*, 1899." In *The Social Survey in Historical Perspective, 1880–1940*, edited by Martin Bulmer, Kevin Bales, and Kathryn Kish Sklar, 170–88. Cambridge: Cambridge University Press, 1991.

Bulmer, Martin, Kevin Bales, and Kathryn Kish Sklar. "The Social Survey in Historical Perspective." In *The Social Survey in Historical Perspective, 1880–1940*, edited by Martin Bulmer, Kevin Bales, and Kathryn Kish Sklar, 1–48. Cambridge: Cambridge University Press, 1991.

———, eds. *The Social Survey in Historical Perspective, 1880–1940*. Cambridge: Cambridge University Press, 1991.

Business Council on Indoor Air. "Building Systems Approach to Indoor Air Quality." Fairfax, Va.: Business Council on Indoor Air, 1994.

"The Business Council on Indoor Air: A Multi-industry Response to an Emerging Public Policy Issue." *Healthy Buildings International Magazine* 1, no. 3 (1991): 6–7.

Butler, Judith. *Bodies That Matter: On the Discursive Limits of "Sex."* New York: Routledge, 1993.

——. "Performativity's Social Magic." In *The Social and Political Body,* edited by Theodore Shatzki and Wolfgang Natter, 29–48. New York: Guilford, 1996.

California Medical Association. "Clinical Ecology: A Critical Appraisal." *Western Journal of Medicine* 144, no. 2 (1986): 239–45.

Carnsdale, J. H. "ASHRAE: A Chronicle of Progress, 1894–1969." *ASHRAE Journal,* June 1969, 47–55.

Carnsdale, James. "KSU Emphasizes Applied Research for Tomorrow's Environment." *ASHRAE Journal,* Nov. 1968, 31–36.

Carrier, W. H. "Committee on Temperature, Humidity and Air Motion." *Transactions* 34 (1928): 23–27.

Carroll, Glenn, ed. *Ecological Models of Organizations.* Cambridge: Ballinger, 1988.

Carson, Rachel. *Silent Spring.* New York: Crest, 1962.

Cassedy, Ellen, and Karen Nussbaum. *9 to 5: The Working Woman's Guide to Office Survival.* New York: Penguin, 1983.

Cassedy, James. *Charles V. Chapin and the Public Health Movement.* Cambridge: Harvard University Press, 1962.

Castells, Manuel. *The Rise of the Network Society.* Cambridge, U.K.: Blackwell, 1996.

Castleman, Barry, and Grace Ziem. "Corporate Influence on Threshold Limit Values." *American Journal of Industrial Medicine* 13 (1988): 531–59.

——. "American Conference of Governmental Industrial Hygienists: Low Threshold of Credibility." *American Journal of Industrial Medicine* 26, no. 1 (1994): 133–43.

Cayleff, Susan. "'She Was Rendered Incapacitated by Menstrual Difficulties': Historical Perspectives on Perceived Intellectual and Physiological Impairment among Menstruating Women." In *Menstrual Health in Women's Lives,* edited by Alice Dan and Linda Lewis, 229–35. Urbana: University of Illinois Press, 1992.

"Charles-Edward Amory Winslow, 1877–1957" (obituary). *ASHRAE Transactions* 63 (1957): 543–44.

Chavkin, Wendy, ed. *Double Exposure: Women's Health Hazards on the Job and at Home.* New York: Monthly Review Press, 1984.

Clark, Claudia. *Radium Girls: Women and Industrial Health Reform, 1910–35.* Chapel Hill: University of North Carolina Press, 1997.

Clark, William. *At War Within: The Double-Edged Sword of Immunity*. New York: Oxford University Press, 1995.

Clarke, Adele. *Disciplining Reproduction: Modernity, American Life Sciences and the Problem of Sex*. Berkeley: University of California Press, 1998.

Cohen, Gary, and John O'Connor, eds. *Fighting Toxics: A Manual for Protecting Your Family, Community, and Workplace*. Washington, D.C.: Island, 1990.

Cohen, Irun. "The Self, the World and Autoimmunity." *Scientific American* 258, no. 4 (1988): 52–60.

Cohen, Steven. "The Pittsburgh Survey and the Social Survey Movement: A Sociological Road Not Taken." In *The Social Survey in Historical Perspective, 1880–1940*, edited by Martin Bulmer, Kevin Bales, and Kathryn Kish Sklar, 245–68. Cambridge: Cambridge University Press, 1991.

College Settlements Association. *Fourth Annual Report of the College Settlements Association from September 1, 1892, to September 1, 1893*. Philadelphia: Avil Printing and Lithographing, 1894.

Colligan, Michael. "The Psychological Effects of Indoor Air Pollution." *Bulletin of the New York Academy of Medicine* 57, no. 10 (1981): 1014–26.

——. "A Review of Mass Psychogenic Illness in Work Settings." In *Mass Psychogenic Illness*, edited by Michael Colligan, James Pennebaker, and Lawrence Murphy, 33–42. Hillsdale, N.J.: Lawrence Erlbaum Associates, 1982.

Colligan, Michael, and Lawrence Murphy. "Mass Psychogenic Illness in Organizations: An Overview." *Journal of Occupational Psychology* 52 (1979).

Collins, Peter. *Changing Ideals in Modern Architecture, 1750–1950*. London: Faber and Faber, 1965.

Consumer Product Safety Commission. "Alert Sheet: Urea Formaldehyde Foam Insulation." Washington, D.C.: U.S. Government Printing Office, 1980.

"Constantine Yaglou, 1896–1960" (obituary). *ASHRAE Journal*, July 1960, 68.

Cooper, Gail. *Air-Conditioning America: Engineers and the Controlled Environment, 1900–1960*. Baltimore: Johns Hopkins University Press, 1998.

Copeland, Douglas. *Generation X: Tales of an Accelerated Culture*. New York: St. Martins, 1991.

Corn, Jacqueline. *Protecting the Health of Workers: The American Conference of Governmental Industrial Hygienists*. Cincinnati: American Conference of Governmental Industrial Hygienists, 1989.

Cowan, Henry. *Science and Building: Structural and Environmental Design in the Nineteenth and Twentieth Centuries*. New York: John Wiley and Sons, 1978.

Cowan, Ruth Schwartz. *More Work for Mother: The Ironies of Household Technology from the Open Hearth to the Microwave*. New York: Basic Books, 1983.

Crary, Jonathan. *Suspensions of Perception: Attention, Spectacle, and Modern Culture*. Cambridge: MIT Press, 1999.

Cullen, Mark, ed. *Workers with Multiple Chemical Sensitivities*. Vol. 2, *Occupational Medicine: State of the Art Reviews*. Philadelphia: Hanley and Belfus, 1987.

Cunningham, James, and Nadja Zalokar. "The Economic Progress of Black Women, 1940–1980: Occupational Distribution and Relative Wages." *Industrial and Labor Relations Review* 45, no. 3 (1992): 540–55.

Daston, Lorraine. "The Coming into Being of Scientific Objects." In *Biographies of Scientific Objects*, edited by Lorraine Daston, 1–14. Chicago: University of Chicago Press, 2000.

Davidow, Ellen Messer. "Acting Otherwise." In *Provoking Agents: Gender and Agency in Theory and Practice*, edited by Judith Keegan Gardner, 23–51. Urbana: University of Illinois Press, 1995.

Davies, Margery. *Women's Place Is at the Typewriter: Office Work and Office Workers, 1870–1930*. Philadelphia: Temple University Press, 1982.

Davis, Audrey. "Life Insurance and the Physical Examination: A Chapter in the Rise of American Medical Technology." *Bulletin of the History of Medicine* 55 (1981): 392–406.

Davis, Susan. "Organizing from Within." *Ms.* 1 (1972): 92–99.

Deleuze, Gilles. "Pensée nomade." In *Nietzsche aujourd'hui*, 159–74. Paris: UGE, 1973.

——. *Foucault*. Translated by Sean Hand. Minneapolis: University of Minnesota Press, 1988.

Deleuze, Gilles, and Claire Parnet. "Many Politics." In *Dialogues*. Translated by Hugh Tomlinson and Barbara Habberjam, 124–47. New York: Columbia University Press, 1977.

Deleuze, Gilles, and Félix Guattari. *A Thousand Plateaus: Capitalism and Schizophrenia*. Translated by Brian Massumi. Minneapolis: University of Minnesota Press, 1987.

Delgado, Alan. *The Enormous File: A Social History of the Office*. London: John Murray, 1979.

Delgado, Richard, and Jean Stefancic, eds. *Critical White Studies: Looking beyond the Mirror*. Philadelphia: Temple University Press, 1997.

DeLillo, Don. *White Noise*. New York: Penguin, 1985.

Dembe, Allard E. *Occupation and Disease: How Social Factors Affect the Conception of Work-Related Disorders*. New Haven, Conn.: Yale University Press, 1996.

Devault, Ileen. *Sons and Daughters of Labor: Class and Clerical Work in Turn-of-the-Century Pittsburgh*. Ithaca, N.Y.: Cornell University Press, 1990.

Di Chiro, Giovanna. "Defining Environmental Justice: Women's Voices and Grassroots Politics." *Socialist Review* 22, no. 4 (1992): 93–130.

——. "Local Actions, Global Visions: Remaking Environmental Expertise." *Frontiers* 18, no. 2 (1997): 203–31.

Dickey, Lawrence, ed. *Clinical Ecology.* Springfield, Ill.: Charles C. Thomas, 1976.

Diller, Elizabeth, and Ricardo Scofidio, eds. *Flesh: Architectural Probes.* New York: Princeton Architectural Press, 1994.

Diner, Steven. "Washington—The Black Majority: Race and Politics in the Nation's Capital." In *Snowbelt Cities: Metropolitan Politics in the Northeast and Midwest since World War II,* edited by Richard M. Bernard, 247–65. Bloomington: Indiana University Press, 1990.

Donaldson, Barry. *Heat and Cold—Mastering the Great Indoors: A Selective History of Heating, Ventilation, Air-Conditioning and Refrigeration from the Ancients to the 1930s.* Atlanta: ASHRAE, 1994.

Donnay, Albert. "MCS or IEI? Depends on W.H.O. You Ask. . . ." Press release, MCS Referral and Resources, March 26, 1996.

Drinker, Philip. "Laboratories of Ventilation and Illumination, Harvard School of Public Health, Boston." *Journal of Industrial Hygiene* 6, no. 1 (1924): 57–66.

Drucker, Peter. *The Ecological Vision: Reflections on the American Condition.* New Brunswick, N.J.: Transaction, 1993.

DuBois, W. E. B. *The Philadelphia Negro.* Philadelphia: University of Pennsylvania, 1899.

——. *The Souls of Black Folk.* Chicago: A. C. McClurg, 1903.

——. *The Autobiography of W. E. B. DuBois.* New York: International, 1968.

Duehring, Cindy. "Carpet, Part One: EPA Stalls and Industry Hedges while Consumers Remain at Risk." *Informed Consent* 1, no. 1 (1993): 6–11, 30–33.

Duehring, Cindy, and Cynthia Wilson. *The Human Consequences of the Chemical Problem.* Sulpher Springs, Mont.: TT Publishing, 1994.

Dumit, Joseph. "Invisible Emerging Illnesses and New Social Movements." Paper presented at the conference "What's New about Emerging Illnesses?," Center for Literary and Cultural Studies, Harvard University. Cambridge, Mass., Nov. 13, 1997.

Dwyer, John. *The Body at War: The Miracle of the Immune System.* New York: New American Library, 1988.

Dyer, Richard. "White." *Screen* 29, no. 4 (1998): 44–65.

Echols, Alice. *Daring to Be Bad: Radical Feminism in America, 1967–75.* Minneapolis: University of Minnesota Press, 1989.

Edwards, J. H., A. J. Griffiths, and J. Mullins. "Protozoa as Sources of Antigen in Humidifier Fever." *Nature* 264 (1976): 438–39.

Ehrenreich, Barbara. *Fear of Falling: The Inner Life of the Middle Class*. New York: Pantheon, 1989.

Eisenberg, David, et al. "Unconventional Medicine in the United States: Prevalence, Costs, and Patterns of Use." *New England Journal of Medicine* 328, no. 4 (1993): 246–52.

Elliot, Cecil. *Technics and Architecture: The Development of Materials and Systems for Buildings*. Cambridge: MIT Press, 1992.

Environmental Action Foundation. *Making Polluters Pay: A Citizens' Guide to Legal Action and Organizing*. Washington, D.C.: Environmental Action Foundation, 1987.

Epstein, Steven. *Impure Science: AIDS, Activism and the Politics of Knowledge*. Berkeley: University of California Press, 1996.

Faust, Halley, and Lawrence Brilliant. "Is the Diagnosis of 'Mass Hysteria' an Excuse for Incomplete Investigation of Low-Level Environmental Contamination?" *Journal of Occupational Medicine* 23, no. 1 (1981): 11–16.

Fee, Elizabeth. *Disease and Discovery: A History of the Johns Hopkins School of Hygiene and Public Health, 1916–39*. Baltimore: Johns Hopkins University Press, 1987.

Feldberg, Roslyn. "'Union Fever': Organizing among Clerical Workers, 1900–1930." *Radical America* 14, no. 3 (1980): 53–70.

Fine, Lisa. *Souls of the Skyscraper: Female Clerical Workers in Chicago, 1870–1930*. Philadelphia: Temple University Press, 1990.

Finnegan, M., and C. Pickering. "Review: Building Related Illness." *Clinical Allergy* 16 (1986): 389–405.

Finnegan, M. J., and C. A. C. Pickering. "Building Related Illness." *Clinical Allergy* 16 (1986): 389–405.

Finnegan, M. J., C. A. C. Pickering, and P. S. Burge. "The Sick Building Syndrome: Prevalence Studies." *British Medical Journal* 209 (1984): 1573–75.

Fischer, Frank. *Citizens, Experts and the Environment: The Politics of Local Knowledge*. Durham, N.C.: Duke University Press, 2000.

Fonda, Jane. *Jane Fonda's Workout Book*. New York: Simon and Schuster, 1981.

Fortun, Kim. *Advocacy after Bhopal*. Chicago: University of Chicago Press, 2000.

Fortun, Mike. "Defining Disease and Health: Multiple Chemical Sensitivity." Unpublished manuscript, 1998.

Forty, Adrian. *Objects of Desire: Design and Society, 1750–1980*. London: Thames and Hudson, 1986.

Foucault, Michel. *The Archaeology of Knowledge; and The Discourse of Language*. Translated by A. M. Sheridan Smith. New York: Harper and Row, 1972.

Foucault, Michel. *The History of Sexuality*. Vol. 1, *An Introduction*. Translated by Robert Hurley. New York: Random House, 1978.

——. *Discipline and Punish: The Birth of the Prison*. Translated by Alan Sheridan. New York: Vintage, 1979.

——. "Technologies of the Self." In *Technologies of the Self: A Seminar with Michel Foucault*, edited by Luther Martin, Huck Gutman, and Patrick Hutton, 16–49. Amherst: University of Massachusetts Press, 1988.

Fowlkes, Martha, and Patricia Miller. "Chemicals and Community at Love Canal." In *The Social and Cultural Construction of Risk*, edited by Branden Johnson and Vincent Covello, 55–80. Dordrecht, the Netherlands: D. Reidel, 1987.

Fox, Steve. *Toxic Work: Women Workers at GTE Lenkurt*. Philadelphia: Temple University Press, 1991.

Fraser, D. W., et al. "Legionnaires' Disease: Description of an Epidemic Pneumonia." *New England Journal of Medicine* 297 (1977): 1189–97.

Freeman, Carla. *High Tech and High Heels in the Global Economy: Women, Work, and Pink-Collar Identities in the Caribbean*. Durham, N.C.: Duke University Press, 2000.

Freeman, John, and Michael Hannan. "The Population Ecology of Organizations." *American Journal of Sociology* 82 (1977): 929–64.

Freeman, Theresa. "Vermonters Organized for Clean-Up." In *Empowering Ourselves: Women and Toxics Organizing*, edited by Robbin Lee Zeff, Marsha Love, and Karen Stults, 42–43. Falls Church, Va.: Center for Health, Environment, and Justice, 1989.

Frumkin, Howard, and Warren Kantrowitz. "Cancer Clusters in the Workplace: An Approach to Investigation." *Journal of Occupational Medicine* 29 (1987): 949–52.

Galbraith, John Kenneth. *The Affluent Society*. Boston: Houghton Mifflin, 1958.

Galison, Peter. "Aufbau/Bauhaus: Logical Positivism and Architectural Modernism." *Critical Inquiry* 16 (1990): 709–52.

——. "The Ontology of the Enemy: Norbert Wiener and the Cybernetic Vision." *Critical Inquiry* 21 (1994): 228–66.

——. *Image and Logic: A Material Culture of Microphysics*. Chicago: University of Chicago Press, 1997.

Galison, Peter, and Lorraine Daston. "The Image of Objectivity." *Representations*, no. 40 (Fall 1992): 81–128.

Garnier, Michael, et al. "Humidifier Lung: An Outbreak in Office Workers." *Chest* 77, no. 2 (1980): 183–87.

Garreau, Joel. *Edge City: Life on the New Frontier*. New York: Doubleday, 1991.

Garrison, Barbara. *The Electronic Sweatshop*. New York: Penguin, 1988.

General Accounting Office. *Siting of Hazardous Waste Landfills and Their*

Correlation with Racial and Economic Status of Surrounding Communities.
Washington, D.C.: GAO/RCED, 1983.

Gibbs, Lois. *Love Canal: My Story.* Albany: State University of New York
Press, 1982.

Gibson, Pamela Reed. "Environmental Illness/Multiple Chemical Sensitivities." *Women and Therapy* 14, no. 3/4 (1993): 171–85.

Gilbert, Ben. *Ten Blocks from the White House: Anatomy of the Washington
Riots of 1968.* New York: Praeger, 1968.

Gillespie, Richard. *Manufacturing Knowledge: A History of the Hawthorne
Experiments.* Cambridge: Cambridge University Press, 1991.

Gillette, Howard, Jr. *Between Justice and Beauty: Race, Planning and the Failure of Urban Policy in Washington, D.C.* Baltimore: Johns Hopkins University Press, 1995.

Glantz, Stan, and S. Aguinaga Bialous. "ASHRAE Standard 62: Tobacco Industry's Influence over National Ventilation Standards." *Tobacco Control*
11 (2002): 315–28.

Glenn, Evelyn Nakano. "From Servitude to Service Work: Historical Con-
tinuities in the Racial Division of Paid Reproductive Labor." *Signs* 18, no. 1
(1992): 1–43.

Glenn, Evelyn Nakano, and Roslyn Feldberg. "Proletarianizing Clerical
Work: Technology and Organizational Control in the Office." In *Case
Studies on the Labor Process,* edited by Andrew Zimbalist, 51–72. New
York: Monthly Review Press, 1979.

Goldberg, Roberta. *Organizing Women Office Workers: Dissatisfaction, Consciousness and Action.* New York: Praeger, 1983.

Gordon, Linda. *Pitied but Not Entitled: Single Mothers and the History of Welfare, 1890–1935.* Cambridge: Harvard University Press, 1994.

Gori, Gio. "The Role of Objective Science in Policy Development." Paper
presented at the symposium "Multiple Chemical Sensitivities: State-of-
the-Science." Baltimore, Oct. 30, 1995.

Gothe, Carl J., Carl M. Odont, and Carl G. Nilsson. "The Environmental
Somatization Syndrome." *Psychosomatics* 36, no. 1 (1995): 1–11.

Gots, Ronald. *Toxic Risks: Science, Regulation, and Perception.* Boca Raton,
Fla.: Lewis, 1992.

——. "Medical Hypothesis and Medical Practice: Autointoxication and Multiple Chemical Sensitivities." *Regulatory Toxicology and Pharmacology* 18
(1993): 2–12.

——. "Multiple Chemical Sensitivities—Public Policy." *Clinical Toxicology* 33,
no. 2 (1995): 111–13.

Green, Venus. *Race on the Line: Gender, Labor and Technology in the Bell
System, 1880–1980.* Durham, N.C.: Duke University Press, 2001.

Greenbaum, Joan. *Windows on the Workplace: Computers, Jobs, and the Orga-*

nization of Office Work in the Late Twentieth Century. New York: Monthly Review Press, 1995.

Greenlee, Edwin J. "Biomedicine and Ideology: A Social History of the Conceptualization and Treatment of Essential Hypertension in the United States." PhD diss., Temple University, 1989.

Greenwood, Judith. "A Historical Perspective on Workers' Compensation in the Context of National Health Policy Debate." In *Workers' Compensation Health Care Cost Containment*, edited by Judith Greenwood and Alfred Taricco, 1–26. Horsham, Penn.: LRP, 1992.

Grossman, Rachel. "Women's Place in the Integrated Circuit." *Radical America* 14 (1980): 29–49.

Guitotti, Tee, Ralph Alexander, and M. Joseph Fedoruk. "Epidemiologic Features That May Distinguish between Building-Associated Illness Outbreaks Due to Chemical Exposure or Psychogenic Origin." *Journal of Occupational Medicine* 29, no. 2 (1987): 148–50.

Gunn, Ronald, and Marilyn Burroughs. "Work Spaces That Work: Designing High Performance Offices." *Futurist*, March/April 1996, 19–24.

Hacking, Ian. *The Taming of Chance*. Cambridge: Cambridge University Press, 1990.

——. *Historical Ontology*. Cambridge: Harvard University Press, 2002.

Hagen, Joel. *An Entangled Bank: The Origins of Ecosystem Ecology*. New Brunswick, N.J.: Rutgers University Press, 1992.

Haigh, Thomas. "The Chromium-Plated Tabulator: Institutionalizing an Electronic Revolution, 1954–1958." *IEEE Annals of the History of Computing* 23, no. 4 (2001): 75–104.

——. "Inventing Information Systems: The Systems Men and the Computer, 1950–1968." *Business History Review* 75, no. 1 (2001): 15–61.

Haldane, J. S. "The Influence of High Air Temperature." *Journal of Hygiene* 5 no. 4 (1905): 494–513.

Hamilton, Alice. *Exploring the Dangerous Traces: The Autobiography of Alice Hamilton*. Boston: Northeastern University Press, 1985 [1943].

Hamlin, Christopher. "Predisposing Causes and Public Health in Early Nineteenth-Century Medical Thought." *Social History of Medicine* 5, no. 1 (1992): 42–71.

Hannan, Michael, and John Freeman. *Organization Ecology*. Cambridge: Harvard University Press, 1989.

Haraway, Donna. "The Biopolitics of Postmodern Bodies: Constitutions of Self in Immune Systems Discourse." In *Simians, Cyborgs, and Women*, 203–30. New York: Routledge, 1991.

——. "A Cyborg Manifesto: Science, Technology, and Socialist-Feminism in the Late Twentieth Century." In *Simians, Cyborgs and Women*, 149–81. New York: Routledge, 1991.

Haraway, Donna. "Situated Knowledges: The Science Question in Feminism and the Privilege of Partial Perspective." In *Simians, Cyborgs and Women*, 183–201. New York: Routledge, 1991.

——. "The Promises of Monsters: A Regenerative Politics for Inappropriate/d Others." In *Cultural Studies*, edited by Lawrence Grossberg, Cary Nelson, and Paula Treichler, 295–337. New York: Routledge, 1992.

Harding, Sandra. "From Feminist Empiricism to Feminist Standpoint Epistemologies." In *The Science Question in Feminism*, 136–62. Ithaca, N.Y.: Cornell University Press, 1986.

Harlow, Sioban. "Function and Dysfunction: A Historical Critique of the Literature on Menstruation and Work." In *Culture, Society, and Menstruation*, edited by Virginia Olesen and Nancy Fugate Woods, 39–51. Washington, D.C.: Hemisphere, 1986.

Harstock, Nancy. "Comment on Hekman's 'Truth and Method: Feminist Standpoint Theory Revisted'—Truth or Justice?" *Signs* 22, no. 3 (1997): 367–73.

Hartmann, Heidi, ed. *Computer Chips and Paper Clips: Technology and Women's Employment*. Washington, D.C.: National Academy Press, 1987.

Harvey, David. *The Condition of Postmodernity*. Cambridge: Blackwell, 1990.

Hasenyager, Bruce. *Managing the Information Ecology*. Westport, Conn.: Quorum, 1996.

Hayden, Dolores. *The Grand Domestic Revolution: A History of Feminist Design for Homes, Neighborhoods and Cities*. Cambridge: MIT Press, 1981.

Haynes, S., and M. Feinleib. "Women, Work and Coronary Heart Disease: Prospective Findings from the Framingham Heart Study." *American Journal of Public Health* 70, no. 2 (1980): 133–41.

Healthy Buildings International. "HBI Experience, 1980–1989." *Healthy Buildings International Magazine* 1, no. 1 (1990): 7.

Heims, Steve Joshua. *Constructing a Social Science for Postwar America: The Cybernetics Group, 1946–53*. Cambridge: MIT Press, 1991.

Henderson, Lawrence. "The Effects of Social Environment (with Elton Mayo)." *Journal of Industrial Hygiene and Toxicology* 18 (1936): 410–16.

Henderson, Yandell, et al. "Physiological Effects of Automobile Exhaust Gas and Standards of Ventilation for Brief Exposures." *Journal of Industrial Hygiene and Toxicology* 3, no. 3 (1921): 79–137.

Hepler, Allison. *Women in Labor: Mothers, Medicine, and Occupational Health in the United States, 1890–1980*. Columbus: Ohio State University Press, 2000.

Hicks, Jeff. "Tight Building Syndrome: When Work Makes You Sick." *Occupational Health and Safety*, no. 53 (Jan. 1984): 51–56.

Higgens-Evenson, R. Rudy. "From Industrial Police to Workmen's Compensation: Public Policy and Industrial Accidents in New York, 1880–1910." *Labor History* 39, no. 4 (1998): 365–80.

Hill, Leonard, et al. "The Influence of the Atmosphere on Our Health and Comfort in Confined and Crowded Spaces." *Smithsonian Miscellaneous Collections* ix, no. 23 (1913).

Hirzy, J. William, and Rufus Morison. "Carpet/4-Psheylcyclohexene Toxicity: The EPA Headquarters Case." In *The Analysis, Communication, and Perception of Risk*, edited by B. J. Garrick and W. C. Gekler, 51–61. New York: Plenum, 1991.

Hodges, G. R., J. N. Fink, and D. P. Schlueter. "Hypersensitivity Pneumonitis Caused by a Contaminated Cool Mist Vaporizer." *Annals of Internal Medicine* 80 (1974): 501–4.

Hoerr, John. *We Can't Eat Prestige: The Women Who Organized Harvard*. Philadelphia: Temple University Press, 1997.

Hounshell, David, and John Kenley Smith. *Science and Corporate Strategy: Du Pont R&D, 1902–1980*. Cambridge: Cambridge University Press, 1988.

Hoy, Suellen. *Chasing Dirt: The American Pursuit of Cleanliness*. New York: Oxford University Press, 1995.

Huginnie, A. Yvette. "Containment and Emancipation: Race, Class, and Gender in the Cold War West." In *The Cold War American West, 1945–89*, edited by Kevin Fernlund, 51–70. Albuquerque: University of New Mexico Press, 1998.

Hull, Gloria T., Patricia Bell, and Barbara Smith. *All the Women Are White, All the Black Are Men, But Some of Us Are Brave: Black Women's Studies*. Old Westbury, N.Y.: Feminist, 1982.

Inaba, Jeffrey. "Corporate Office Design in Suburbia: The Connecticut General Life Insurance Headquarters." Unpublished manuscript, 1997.

Ingles, Margaret. *Willis Haviland Carrier, Father of Air Conditioning*. Garden City, N.Y.: Country Life, 1952.

Jackson, Kenneth. *Crabgrass Frontier: The Suburbanization of the United States*. Oxford: Oxford University Press, 1987.

Jain, Sarah. "Inscription Fantasies and Interface Erotics: A Social-Material Analysis of Keyboards, Repetitive Strain Injuries and Products Liability Law." *Hastings Women's Law Journal* 9, no. 2 (1998): 219–53.

Jameson, Fredric. *Postmodernism, or, The Cultural Logic of Late Capitalism*. Durham, N.C.: Duke University Press, 1991.

Janssen, John. "The V in ASHRAE: An Historical Perspective." *ASHRAE Journal*, Aug. 1994, 126–32.

Jaret, Peter. "Our Immune System: The Wars Within." *National Geographic*, June 1986, 702–5.

Jasanoff, Sheila. "Science, Politics, and the Renegotiation of Expertise at EPA." *Osiris* 7, no. 2 (1992): 195–217.

——. *Science at the Bar: Law, Science, and Technology*. Cambridge: Harvard University Press, 1995.

Johnson, Philip, and Henry Russel Hitchcock. *The International Style: Architecture since 1922*. New York: MOMA, 1932.

Jones, Beverly W. "Before Montgomery and Greensboro: The Desegregation Movement in the District of Columbia, 1950–1953." *Phylon* 43 (1982): 144–54.

Jordy, William H. "The Aftermath of the Bauhaus in America: Gropius, Mies, and Breuer." In *The Intellectual Migration: Europe and America, 1930–1960*, edited by Donald Fleming and Bernard Bailyn, 485–543. Cambridge: Harvard University Press, 1969.

Judkins, Bennett. *We Offer Ourselves as Evidence: Toward Workers' Control of Occupational Health*. New York: Greenwood, 1986.

Kates, Carol. "Working Class Feminism and Feminist Unions: Title VII, the UAW and NOW." *Labor Studies Journal* 14 (1989): 28–45.

Katz, Michael, and Thomas Sugrue. *W. E. B. DuBois, Race, and the City: "The Philadelphia Negro" and Its Legacy*. Philadelphia: University of Pennsylvania Press, 1998.

Kelley, Florence. "Hull House." *New England Magazine*, July 1898: 550–66.

Kerckhoff, Alan, and Kurt Back. *The June Bug: A Study of Hysterical Contagion*. New York: Appleton-Century-Crofts, 1968.

Kirsch, Scott. "Harold Knapp and the Geography of Normal Controversy: Radiodine in the Historical Environment." In "Landscapes of Exposure: Knowledge and Illness in Modern Environments," edited by Gregg Mitman, Michelle Murphy, and Christopher Sellers, special issue, *Osiris*, 167–82. Chicago: University of Chicago Press, 2004.

Kleeman, Walter B. *Interior Design of the Electronic Office: The Comfort and Productivity Payoff*. New York: Van Nostrand Reinhold, 1991.

Klein, Judy. *Office Book*. New York: Facts on File, 1982.

Kofie, Nelson. *Race, Class, and the Struggle for Neighborhood in Washington, D.C.* New York: Garland, 1999.

Kohler, Robert. "Medical Reform and Biomedical Science: Biochemistry—a Case Study." In *The Therapeutic Revolution: Essays in the Social History of American Medicine*, edited by Morris Vogel and Charles Rosenberg, 27–66. Philadelphia: University of Pennsylvania, 1979.

Kosterlitz, Julie. "Luring Women to Labor's Ranks." *National Journal*, March 15, 1997, 541.

Krauss, Celene. "Blue-Collar Women and Toxic-Waste Protests: The Process of Politicization." In *Toxic Struggles: The Theory and Practice of Environmental Justice*, edited by Richard Hofrichter, 107–17. Philadelphia: New Society, 1993.

——. "Women and Toxic Waste Protests: Race, Class, and Gender as Resources of Resistance." *Qualitative Sociology* 16, no. 3 (1993): 247–62.

——. "Challenging Power: Toxic Waste Protests and the Politicization of

White Working-Class Women." In *Community Activism and Feminist Politics: Organizing across Race, Class and Gender,* edited by Nancy Naples, 129–50. New York: Routledge, 1998.

Kristeva, Julia. *Powers of Horror: An Essay on Abjection.* Translated by Leon Roudiez. New York: Columbia University Press, 1982.

Kroll-Smith, Steve, and H. Hugh Floyd. *Bodies in Protest: Environmental Illness and the Struggle over Medical Knowledge.* New York: New York University Press, 1997.

Kugelmann, Robert. *Stress: The Nature and History of Engineered Grief.* Westport, Conn.: Praeger, 1992.

Kwolek-Folland, Angela. *Engendering Business: Men and Women in the Corporate Office, 1870–1930.* Baltimore: Johns Hopkins University Press, 1994.

Land, Marc, Marc Roberts, and Stephen Thomas. *The Environmental Protection Agency: Asking the Wrong Questions.* New York: Oxford University Press, 1990.

Lasch-Quinn, Elizabeth. *Black Neighbors: Race and the Limits of Reform in the American Settlement Movement, 1890–1945.* Chapel Hill: University of North Carolina Press, 1993.

Lash, Johnathon, Katherine Gillman, and David Sheridan. *A Season of Spoils: The Story of the Reagan Administration's Attack on the Environment.* New York: Pantheon, 1984.

Latour, Bruno. *The Pasteurization of France.* Cambridge: Harvard University Press, 1988.

——. "Mixing Humans and Nonhumans Together: The Sociology of a Door-Closer." *Social Problems* 35, no. 3 (1998): 298–310.

Lavelle, M., and N. Coyle. "A Special Investigation; Unequal Protection: The Racial Divide in Environmental Law." *National Law Journal* (1992): S1–S16.

Law, John, and Annemarie Mol. "Notes on Materiality and Sociality." *Sociological Review* 43 (1995): 274–94.

——, eds. *Complexities: Social Studies of Knowledge Practices.* Durham, N.C.: Duke University Press, 2002.

Lawson, Lynn. *Staying Well in a Toxic World.* Chicago: Noble, 1993.

Le Corbusier. *Précisions.* Paris: G. Crès, 1930.

Leffingwell, William. *Office Management: Principles and Practice.* Chicago: A. W. Shaw, 1927.

Leffingwell, William H. *Scientific Office Management.* Chicago: A. W. Shaw, 1917.

——. *The Office Appliance Manual.* Chicago: National Association of Office Appliance Manufacturers, 1926.

Legator, Marvin, Barbara Harper, and Michael Schott, eds. *The Health Detectives Handbook: A Guide to the Investigation of Environmental Health Hazards.* Baltimore: Johns Hopkins University Press, 1985.

Levin, Hal. "Building Ecology." *Progressive Architecture*, April 1981, 173–75.

——. "Healthy Buildings, Where Do We Stand? Where Should We Go?" In *Chemical, Microbiological, Health, and Comfort Aspects of Indoor Air Quality—State of the Art in sbs*, edited by Helmut Knöpple and Peter Wolkoff, 361–71. Dordrecht, the Netherlands: Kluwer Academic, 1992.

Levin, Hal, and Kevin Teichman. "Indoor Air Quality—For Architects." *Progressive Architecture*, March 1991, 52–57.

Levin, Myron. "Who's Behind the Building Doctor?" *Nation*, Aug. 9, 1993, 168–71.

Levine, Adeline G. *Love Canal: Science, Politics, and People*. Lexington, Mass.: Heath, 1982.

Light, Jennifer. "When Computers Were Women." *Technology and Culture* 4, no. 3 (1999): 455–83.

Lapartito, Kenneth. "When Women Were Switches: Technology, Work, and Gender in the Telephone Industry, 1890–1920." *American Historical Review* 99 (1994): 1075–1111.

Lipsitz, George. *The Possessive Investment in Whiteness: How White People Profit from Identity Politics*. Philadelphia: Temple University Press, 1998.

Locke, Margaret. *Twice Dead: Organ Transplants and the Reinvention of Death*. Berkeley: University of California Press, 2002.

Lofroth, Gören, Edward Hefner, Ingrid Alfheim, and Mona Moeller. "Mutagenic Activity in Photocopies." *Science*, Aug. 29, 1980, 1037–39.

Lukács, Georg. "Reification and the Consciousness of the Proletariat." In *History and Class Consciousness*, 83–222. London: Merlin Press, 1971.

Lupton, Ellen. *Mechanical Brides: Women and Machines from Home to Office*. Princeton, N.J.: Princeton Architectural Press, 1993.

Mahoney, Martha. "Residential Segregation and White Privilege." In *Critical White Studies: Looking beyond the Mirror*, edited by Richard Delgado and Jean Stefancic, 273–76. Philadelphia: Temple University Press, 1997.

Makower, Joel. *Office Hazards: How Your Job Can Make You Sick*. Washington, D.C.: Tilden, 1981.

Mandell, Nikki. *The Corporation as Family: The Gendering of Corporate Welfare, 1890–1930*. Chapel Hill: University of North Carolina Press, 2002.

Manning, Robert. "Multicultural Washington, D.C.: The Changing Social and Economic Landscape of a Post-industrial Metropolis." *Ethnic and Racial Studies* 21, no. 2 (1998): 328–55.

Markowitz, Gerald, and David Rosner. "The Limits of Thresholds: Silica and the Politics of Science, 1935–1990." *American Journal of Public Health* 85, no. 2 (1995): 253–62.

Marschall, Daniel, and Judith Gregory, eds. *Office Automation, Jekyll or Hyde? Highlights of the International Conference on Office Work and New Technology*. Cleveland: Working Women Education Fund, 1983.

Martin, Emily. *The Woman in the Body*. Boston: Beacon, 1989.

——. *Flexible Bodies*. Boston: Beacon, 1993.

Martin, James. *Cybercorp: The New Business Revolution*. New York: AMACOM, 1996.

Massachusetts History Workshop. *They Can't Run the Office without Us: Sixty Years of Clerical Work*. Cambridge: Massachusetts History Workshop, 1985.

Massumi, Brian. *A User's Guide to Capitalism and Schizophrenia: Deviations from Deleuze and Guattari*. Cambridge: MIT Press, 1993.

Mazur, Allan. *A Hazardous Inquiry: The Rashomon Effect at Love Canal*. Cambridge: Harvard University Press, 1998.

McIntosh, Robert. *The Background of Ecology*. Cambridge: Cambridge University Press, 1985.

Meikle, Jeffrey. *American Plastic: A Cultural History*. New Brunswick, N.J.: Rutgers University Press, 1995.

Melucci, Alberto. *Nomads of the Present: Social Movements and Individual Needs in Contemporary Society*. Translated by John Keane and Paul Mier. Philadelphia: Temple University Press, 1989.

——. *Challenging Codes: Collective Action in the Information Age*. Cambridge: Cambridge University Press, 1996.

Messing, Karen, and Donna Mergler. " 'The Rat Couldn't Speak, but We Can': Inhumanity in Occupational Health Research." In *Reinventing Biology: Respect for Life and the Creation of Knowledge*, edited by Lynda Birke and Ruth Hubbard, 21–49. Bloomington: Indiana University Press, 1995.

Milgrome, Harry. *The Adventure Book of Weather*. New York: Capital, 1959.

Mills, C. Wright. *White Collar*. New York: Oxford University Press, 1953.

Mintz, Mortin. "Smoke Screen." *Washington Post Magazine*, March 24, 1996, 12–30.

Mitman, Gregg. *The State of Nature: Ecology, Community and American Social Thought*. Chicago: University of Chicago Press, 1992.

Mitman, Gregg, Michelle Murphy, and Christopher Sellers. "Introduction: A Cloud over History." In "Landscapes of Exposure: Knowledge and Illness in Modern Environments," edited by Gregg Mitman, Michelle Murphy, and Christopher Sellers, special issue, *Osiris*, 1–17. Chicago: University of Chicago Press, 2004.

Mohanty, Chandra. "Feminist Encounters: Locating the Politics of Experience." *Copyright* 1 (1987): 30–44.

Mol, Annemarie. *The Body Multiple: Ontology in Medical Practice*. Durham, N.C.: Duke University Press, 2003.

Montague, Peter. "Our Stolen Future: Part 2." *Rachel's Environment and Health Weekly*, no. 487 (March 28, 1996).

Moore, James. *The Death of Competition: Leadership and Strategy in the Age of Business Ecosystems*. New York: Harper Business, 1996.

Morawski, Jill. "White Experimenters, White Blood, and Other White Conditions: Locating the Psychologist's Race." In *Off White: Readings on Race, Power, and Society*, edited by Michelle Fine et al., 13–28. New York: Routledge, 1997.

Moss, David. "Kindling a Flame under Federalism: Progressive Reformers, Corporate Elites, and the Phosphorus Poisoning Campaign of 1909–12." *Business History Review* 68 (1994): 244–75.

Murphy, Michelle. "Hearing Gulf War Syndrome." Unpublished manuscript, 1996.

——. "Immodest Witnessing: The Epistemology of Vaginal Self-Examination in the U.S. Feminist Self-Help Movement." *Feminist Studies* 30 (2004): 115–47.

Murray, Thomas. "Regulating Asbestos: Ethics, Politics and the Values of Science." In *The Health and Safety of Workers*, edited by Ronald Bayer, 271–92. New York: Oxford University Press, 1988.

Naismith, Gaye. "Tales from the Crypt: Contamination and Quarantine in Todd Haynes' *Safe*." In *The Visible Woman: Imaging Technologies, Gender and Science*, edited by Lisa Cartwright, 360–87. New York: New York University Press, 1997.

Nash, Linda. "The Fruits of Ill-Health: Pesticides and Workers' Bodies in Post–World War II California." In "Landscapes of Exposure: Knowledge and Illness in Modern Environments," edited by Gregg Mitman, Michelle Murphy, and Christopher Sellers, special issue, *Osiris*, 203–19. Chicago: University of Chicago Press, 2004.

National Commission on State Workmen's Compensation Laws. *The Report of the National Commission on State Workmen's Compensation Laws*. Washington, D.C.: U.S. Government Printing Office, 1972.

Nelkin, Dorothy, and Michael Brown. *Workers at Risk: Voices for the Workplace*. Chicago: University of Chicago Press, 1984.

Nelson, Daniel. *Fredrick W. Taylor and the Rise of the New Factory System*. Madison: University of Wisconsin Press, 1980.

Newman, Penny. "Killing Legally with Toxic Waste: Women and the Environment in the United States." In *Close to Home: Women Reconnect Ecology, Health and Development Worldwide*, edited by Vandana Shiva, 43–59. Philadelphia: New Society, 1994.

New York State Commission on Ventilation. *Ventilation: Report of the New York State Commission on Ventilation*. New York: E. P. Dutton, 1923.

Nilsson, Lennart. *The Body Victorious: The Illustrated Story of Our Immune System and Other Defenses of the Human Body*. New York: Delacorte, 1987.

9to5. *The 9to5 National Survey on Women and Stress*. Cleveland: 9to5, National Association of Working Women, 1984.

9to5. *Hidden Victims: Clerical Workers, Automation, and the Changing Economy.* Cleveland: Working Women, 1985.

———. *VDT Syndrome: The Physical and Mental Trauma of Computer Work.* Cleveland: Working Women, 1988.

Nugent, Angela. "Fit for Work: The Introduction of Physical Examinations in Industry." *Bulletin of the History of Medicine* 57 (1983): 578–95.

Nussbaum, Karen. "Office Automation: Jekyll or Hyde?" In *Office Automation: Jekyll or Hyde?*, edited by Daniel Marschall and Judith Gregory, 16–19. Cleveland: Working Women Education Fund, 1983.

Odum, Eugene. *Fundamentals of Ecology.* 3rd ed. Philadelphia: W. B. Saunders, 1971.

———. *Ecology: The Link between the Natural and Social Sciences.* 2nd ed. New York: Holt, Rinehart and Winston, 1975.

———. "The Emergence of Ecology as a New Integrative Discipline." *Science* 195 (1977): 1289.

Odum, H. T. "Ecological Potential and Analogue Circuits for the Ecosystem." *American Scientist* 48 (1960): 1–8.

Odum, Howard. *Environment, Power and Society.* New York: Wiley Interscience, 1971.

Oldenziel, Ruth. *Making Technology Masculine: Men, Women and Modern Machines in America, 1870–1945.* Amsterdam: Amsterdam University Press, 1999.

O'Mahoney, M., et al. "Legionnaires' Disease and the Sick-Building Syndrome." *Epidemiology and Infection* 103 (1989): 285–92.

Ong, Aihwa. *Spirits of Resistance and Capitalist Discipline: Factor Women in Malaysia.* Albany: SUNY Press, 1987.

Ozonoff, David. "Failed Warnings: Asbestos-Related Disease and Industrial Medicine." In *The Health and Safety of Workers*, edited by Ronald Bayer, 139–218. New York: Oxford University Press, 1988.

Paull, Jeffrey. "The Origin and Basis of Threshold Limit Values." *American Journal of Industrial Medicine* 5, no. 227–38 (1984).

Petersen, Andrea. "Metaphor of a Corporate Display: 'You Work, and Then You Die.'" *Wall Street Journal*, Nov. 8, 1996.

Petryna, Adriana. *Life Exposed: Biological Citizens after Chernobyl.* Princeton, N.J.: Princeton University Press, 2002.

Pile, John. *Open Office Planning.* New York: Whitney Library of Design, 1978.

———. *Open Office Space.* New York: Facts on File, 1984.

Plotke, David, and Karen Nussbaum. "Women Clerical Workers and Trade Unionism: Interview with Karen Nussbaum." *Socialist Review* 49, no. 10 (1980).

Porter, Theodore. *Trust in Numbers: The Pursuit of Objectivity in Science and Public Life.* Princeton, N.J.: Princeton University Press, 1995.

Pouchelle, Marie-Christine. *The Body and Surgery in the Middle Ages.* Translated by Rosemary Morris. Cambridge: Polity, 1983.

Price, Matt. "Body and Soul: The Rehabilitation of Soldiers in the Great War." PhD diss., Stanford University, 1998.

Proctor, Robert. *Cancer Wars: How Politics Shapes What We Know and Don't Know about Cancer.* New York: Basic Books, 1995.

Propst, Robert. *The Office: A Facility Based on Change.* Zeeland, Mich.: Herman Miller, 1968.

Pulgram, William, and Richard Stonis. *Designing the Automated Office.* New York: Whitney Library of Design, 1984.

Rabinbach, Anson. *The Human Motor.* Berkeley: University of California Press, 1990.

Rajapakse, N., E. Silva, and A. Kortenkamp. "Combining Xenoestrogens at Levels below Individual No-Observed-Effect Concentrations Dramatically Enhances Steroid Hormone Action." *Environmental Health Perspectives* 110, no. 9 (2002): 917–21.

Randolph, Theron. "Both Allergy and Clinical Ecology Are Needed." *Annals of Allergy* 39 (1977): 215–16.

———. *Environmental Medicine: Beginnings and Bibliographies of Clinical Ecology.* Fort Collins, Colo.: Clinical Ecology, 1987.

Rasmussen, Brigit Brander, Erick Klinenberg, Irene Nexica, and Matt Wray, eds. *The Making and Unmaking of Whiteness.* Durham, N.C.: Duke University Press, 2001.

Rea, William J., Gerald H. Ross, Alfred R. Johnson, Ralph E. Smiley, Donald E. Sprague, Ervin J. Fenyves, and N. Samadi. "Confirmation of Chemical Sensitivity by Means of Double-Blind Inhalant Challenge of Toxic Volatile Chemicals." *Clinical Ecology* 6, no. 3 (1989): 113–18.

Rea, William J., Gerald H. Ross, Alfred R. Johnson, Ralph E. Smiley, and Ervin J. Fenyves. "Chemical Sensitivity in Physicians." *Clinical Ecology* 6, no. 4 (1989): 135–41.

Rea, William J., Alfred R. Johnson, Gerald H. Ross, Joel R. Butler, Ervin J. Fenyves, Bertie Griffiths, and John Laseter. "Considerations for the Diagnosis of Chemical Sensitivity." In *Multiple Chemical Sensitivity: Addendum to Biologic Markers in Immunotoxicology.* Washington, D.C.: National Academy Press, 1992.

Roach, S. A., and S. M. Rappaport. "But They Are Not Thresholds: A Critical Analysis of the Documentation of Threshold Limit Values." *American Journal of Industrial Medicine* 17, no. 6 (1990): 717–53.

Rogers, Sherry. *Tired or Toxic? A Blueprint for Health.* Syracuse, N.Y.: Prestige, 1990.

Rosen, George. "Politics and Public Health in New York City." *Bulletin of the History of Medicine* 24 (1950): 441–61.

Rosenkrantz, Barbara Gutmann. *Public Health and the State: Changing Views in Massachusetts, 1842–1936.* Cambridge: Harvard University Press, 1972.

Rosner, David, and Gerald Markowitz. *Deadly Dust: Silicosis and the Politics of Occupational Disease in Twentieth-Century America.* Princeton, N.J.: Princeton University Press, 1991.

——. *Deceit and Denial: The Deadly Politics of Industrial Pollution.* Berkeley: University of California Press, 2003.

——, eds. *Dying for Work: Workers' Safety and Health in Twentieth-Century America.* Bloomington: Indiana University Press, 1987.

Rotella, Elyce. *From Home to Office: U.S. Women at Work, 1870–1930.* Ann Arbor: UMI Research Press, 1981.

Rothman, Allan, and Michael Weintraub. "The Sick Building Syndrome and Mass Hysteria." *Neurologic Clinics* 13, no. 2 (1995): 405–12.

Rush, J. E. "A Rational Basis for Ventilation." *ASHVE Transactions* 32 (1926): 321–56.

Ryan, Christopher, and Lisa Morrow. "Dysfunctional Buildings or Dysfunctional People: An Examination of the Sick Building Syndrome and Allied Disorders." *Journal of Consulting and Clinical Psychology* 60, no. 2 (1992): 220–24.

Sacks, Karen Brodkin. "The G.I. Bill: Whites Only Need Apply." In *Critical White Studies: Looking beyond the Mirror,* edited by Richard Delgado and Jean Stefancic, 310–13. Philadelphia: Temple University Press, 1997.

Sandweiss, Stephen. "The Social Construction of Environmental Justice." In *Environmental Injustices, Political Struggles: Race, Class and the Environment,* edited by David Camacho, 31–57. Durham, N.C.: Duke University Press, 1998.

Sanjour, William. "EPA's Revolving Door." *Sierra Magazine,* Sept./Oct. 1992, 77.

Sansbury, Gail Gregory. " 'Now What's the Matter with You Girls?' Clerical Workers Organize." *Radical America* 14 (1980): 67–75.

Sarachild, Kathie. "Consciousness-Raising: A Radical Weapon." In *Feminist Revolution,* edited by Redstockings, 144–50. New Paltz, N.Y.: Redstockings, 1975.

Schlesinger, Hilde. "Letter from Our President, on 'Belonging.' " *New Reactor,* Nov./Dec. 1994, 1.

Schmitt, Neal, Michael Colligan, and Michael Fitzgerald. "Unexplained Physical Symptoms in Eight Organizations: Individual and Organizational Analyses." *Journal of Occupational Psychology* 53, no. 4 (1980): 305–17.

Schneirov, Matthew, and Jonathan David Geczik. "A Diagnosis for Our Times: Alternative Health's Submerged Networks and the Transformation of Identities." *Sociological Quarterly* 37, no. 4 (1996): 627–44.

Scott, Joan W. " 'Experience.' " In *Feminists Theorize the Political*, edited by Joan W. Scott and Judith Butler, 22–40. New York: Routledge, 1995.

Seifer, Nancy, and Barbara Wertheimer. "New Approaches to Collective Power: Four Working Women's Organizations." In *Women Organizing: An Anthology*, 152–83. Metuchen, N.J.: Scarecrow, 1979.

Sellers, Christopher. "Factory as Environment: Industrial Hygiene, Professional Collaboration and the Modern Sciences of Pollution." *Environmental History Review* 18, no. 1 (1994): 55–83.

———. *Hazards of the Job: From Industrial Disease to Environmental Health Science*. Chapel Hill: University of North Carolina Press, 1997.

Seltzer, Mark. *Bodies and Machines*. New York: Routledge, 1992.

Selye, Hans. *The Stress of Life*. New York: McGraw-Hill, 1965.

Sennet, Richard. *Flesh and Stone: The Body and the City in Western Civilization*. New York: W. W. Norton, 1994.

Shapin, Steven, and Simon Schaffer. *Leviathan and the Air-Pump: Hobbes, Boyle and the Experimental Life*. Princeton, N.J.: Princeton University Press, 1989.

Sheehan, Helen E., and Richard P. Wedeen, eds. *Toxic Circles: Environmental Hazards from the Workplace into the Community*. New Brunswick, N.J.: Rutgers University Press, 1993.

Shorter, Edward. *From Paralysis to Fatigue: A History of Psychosomatic Illness in the Modern Era*. New York: Free Press, 1992.

———. *From the Mind into the Body: The Cultural Origins of Psychosomatic Symptoms*. New York: Free Press, 1994.

———. "The Borderland between Neurology and History." *Neurologic Clinics* 13, no. 2 (1995): 229–39.

Shoshkes, Lila. *Space Planning: Designing the Office Environment*. New York: Architectural Record Books, 1976.

Showalter, Elaine. *Hystories: Hysterical Epidemics and Modern Culture*. New York: Columbia University Press, 1997.

Shreve, Anita. *Women Together, Women Alone: The Legacy of the Consciousness-Raising Movement*. New York: Viking, 1989.

Sicherman, Barbara. *Alice Hamilton: A Life in Letters*. Cambridge: Harvard University Press, 1984.

Silverberg, Helene, ed. *Gender and American Social Science*. Princeton, N.J.: Princeton University Press, 1998.

Simon, Gregory E., Wayne J. Katon, and Patrician Sparks. "Allergic to Life: Psychological Factors in Environmental Illness." *American Journal of Psychiatry* 147, no. 7 (1990): 901–6.

Sinclair-Holbrook, Agnes. "Map Notes and Comments." In *Hull-House Maps and Papers: A Presentation of Nationalities and Wages in a Congested District of Chicago Together with Comments and Essays on Problems Growing*

Out of the Social Conditions, edited by Residents of Hull-House, 3–26. New York: Thomas Y. Crowell, 1895.

Singer, Jerome, Carlene Baum, Andrew Baum, and Brenda Thew. "Mass Psychogenic Illness: The Case for Social Comparison." In *Mass Psychogenic Illness,* edited by Michael Colligan, James Pennebaker, and Lawrence Murphy, 155–69. Hillsdale, N.J.: Lawrence Erlbaum Associates, Inc., 1982.

Singhvi, R., R. D. Turpin, and S. M. Burchette. "A Final Summary Report on the Indoor Air Monitoring Performed at USEPA Headquarters, Washington, D.C., on March 4 and 5, 1988." Edison, N.J.: Environmental Protection Agency, 1988.

Sklar, Kathryn Kish. "Hull-House Maps and Papers: Social Science as Women's Work in the 1890s." In *The Social Survey in Historical Perspective, 1880–1940,* edited by Martin Bulmer, Kevin Bales, and Kathryn Kish Sklar, 111–47. Cambridge: Cambridge University Press, 1991.

Smith, Barbara Ellen. *Digging Our Own Graves: Coal Miners and the Struggle over Black Lung Disease.* Philadelphia: Temple University Press, 1987.

Smith, M. G. *Potential Health Hazards of Video Display Terminals.* Cincinnati: NIOSH, June 1981.

Spears, Ellen. "Environmental Justice in Newtown, Georgia." In *Emerging Illnesses and Society: Negotiating the Public Health Agenda,* edited by Randall Packard, 171–90. Baltimore: Johns Hopkins University Press, 2004.

Spivak, Gayatri Chakravorty. *The Post-colonial Critic.* New York: Routledge, 1990.

——. "In a Word: Interview." In *Outside in the Teaching Machine,* 1–23. New York: Routledge, 1993.

Stadler, J. C., et al. "Evaluation of a Method Used to Test for Potential Toxicity of Carpet Emissions." *Food and Chemical Toxicology* 32, no. 11 (1994): 1073–87.

Stafford, Barbara. *Body Criticism: Imaging the Unseen in Enlightenment Art and Medicine.* Cambridge: MIT Press, 1991.

Stahl, Sidney, and Morty Legedun. "Mystery Gas: An Analysis of Mass Hysteria." *Journal of Health and Social Behavior* 15, March (1974): 44–50.

Staudenmayer, Herman, and John Selner. "Failure to Assess Psychopathology in Patients Presenting with Chemical Sensitivities." *Journal of Environmental Medicine* 37, no. 6 (1995): 704–9.

Staudenmayer, Herman, John Selner, and Martin Buhr. "Double-Blind Provacation Chamber Challenges in Twenty Patients Presenting with 'Multiple Chemical Sensitivities.'" *Regulatory Toxicology and Pharmacology* 18, no. 1 (1993): 44–53.

Steele, Fritz. *Making and Managing High-Quality Workplaces: An Organization Ecology.* New York: Teachers College Press, 1986.

Stellman, Jeanne. *Women's Work, Women's Health: Myths and Realities.* New York: Pantheon, 1977.

Stellman, Jeanne, and Mary Sue Henifin. *Office Work Can Be Dangerous to Your Health.* New York: Pantheon, 1983.

Stolwijk, J. A. "Sick Building Syndrome." In *Indoor Air,* edited by B. Berglund, T. Linvall, and J. Sundell, 22–29. Stockholm: Swedish Council for Building Research, 1984.

——. "Sick-Building Syndrome." *Environmental Health Perspectives* 95 (1991): 99–100.

Strom, Sharon Hartman. "'We're No Kitty Foyles': Organizing Office Workers for the Congress of Industrial Organizations, 1937–1950." In *Women, Work and Protest: A Century of U.S. Women's Labor History,* edited by Ruth Milkman, 206–34. Boston: Routledge and Keegan Paul, 1985.

——. *Beyond the Typewriter: Gender, Class, and the Origins of Modern American Office Work, 1900–1930.* Urbana: University of Illinois Press, 1992.

Taylor, Peter. "Technocratic Optimism, H. T. Odum and the Partial Transformation of Ecological Metaphor after World War II." *Journal of the History of Biology* 21, no. 2 (1988): 213–44.

Tchudi, Stephen. "Lesson Plan on Indoor Air Quality." *EPA Journal,* Oct./ Dec. 1993: 42–43.

Tepperman, Jean. *Sixty Words a Minute, and What Do You Get? Clerical Workers Today.* Somerville, Mass.: New England Free Press, 1972.

——. *Not Servants, Not Machines: Office Workers Speak Out.* Boston: Beacon, 1976.

Terr, Abba I. "Environmental Illness: A Clinical Review of Fifty Cases." *Archives in Internal Medicine* 146 (Jan. 1986): 145–49.

——. "'Multiple Chemical Sensitivities': Immunologic Critique of Clinical Ecology Theories and Practice." In *Workers with Multiple Chemical Sensitivities,* edited by Mark Cullen, 683–94. Philadelphia: Hanley and Belfus, 1987.

Thompson, Emily. *The Soundscape of Modernity: Architectural Acoustics and the Culture of Listening in America, 1900–1933.* Cambridge: MIT Press, 2002.

Thompson, Paul, and David McHugh. *Work Organizations: A Critical Introduction.* London: Macmillan, 1990.

Tomes, Nancy. *The Gospel of Germs: Men, Women, and the Microbe in American Life.* Cambridge: Harvard University Press, 1998.

Trinh T. Minh-Ha. *Woman, Native, Other.* Bloomington: Indiana University Press, 1989.

Turiel, Isaac, C. D. Hollowell, R. R. Miksch, J. V. Rudy, and R. A. Young. "The Effects of Reduced Ventilation on Indoor Air Quality in an Office Building." *Atmospheric Environment* 17, no. 1 (1983): 51–64.

U.S. Centers for Disease Control and Prevention. *Second National Report on Human Exposure to Environmental Chemicals*. Atlanta: Centers for Disease Control, 2003.

U.S. Environmental Protection Agency. *The Inside Story*. Washington, D.C.: Environmental Protection Agency, 1988.

———. *Indoor Air Facts No. 5: Environmental Tobacco Smoke*. Washington, D.C.: Office of Air and Radiation, 1989.

———. *Indoor Air Quality and Work Environment Study*, vols. 1–4. Washington, D.C.: Environmental Protection Agency, 1989, 1990, 1991.

———. *Affirmative Program Plan for Women and Minorities: FY 2002 Plan Update and FY 2001 Accomplishment Report*. Washington, D.C.: Environmental Protection Agency, April 2002.

U.S. Environmental Protection Agency and National Institute of Occupational Safety and Health. *Building Air Quality: A Guide for Building Owners and Facility Managers*. Washington, D.C.: U.S. Government Printing Office, 1991.

U.S. Senate Banking Committee. "Senator Gramm's Letter to Acting SEC Chairman Laura Unger Regarding SEC Plan to Move Headquarters." Press release, July 19, 2001.

United Church of Christ Commission on Racial Justice. *Toxic Wastes and Race in the United States*. New York: United Church of Christ, 1987.

Verran, Helen. *Science and an African Logic*. Chicago: University of Chicago Press, 2002.

Vischer, Jacqueline. *Environmental Qualities in Offices*. New York: Van Nostrand Reinhold, 1989.

Viseltear, Arthur. "C.-E. A. Winslow: His Era and His Contribution to Medical Care." In *Healing and History*, edited by Charles Rosenberg, 205–28. New York: Science History, 1979.

Vukelich, Dan. "Employees Charge EPA's Own House Needs Cleaning Up." *Washington Times*, April 28, 1988.

Waldman, Amy. "Labor's New Face." *Nation*, September 22, 1997, 11–16.

Walker, Anne. "A History of Menstrual Psychology." In *The Menstrual Cycle*, 30–58. London: Routledge, 1997.

Wallace, Lance. *The Total Exposure Assessment Methodology (TEAM) Study: Summary and Analysis*, vol. 1. Washington, D.C.: Environmental Protection Agency, 1987.

———. "Preliminary Analysis of the Essay Question." Unpublished manuscript, 1991.

———. "The TEAM Studies." *EPA Journal* 19, no. 4 (1993): 23–24.

Wallingford, Kenneth. *NIOSH IEQ Health Hazard Evaluation Requests*. Cincinnati: IEQ Research Coordinator, 1995.

Waring, Stephen P. *Taylorism Transformed: Scientific Management Theory since 1945*. Chapel Hill: University of North Carolina Press, 1991.

Warren, Christian. *Brushes with Death: A Social History of Lead Poisoning.* Baltimore: Johns Hopkins University Press, 2001.

Watney, Simon. *Policing Desire: Pornography, AIDS, and the Media.* London: Metheun, 1987.

Weindling, Paul, ed. *The Social History of Occupational Health.* London: Croom Helm, 1985.

Weiss, N. S., and Y. Solemanyi. "Hypersensitivity Lung Disease Caused by Contamination of an Air Conditioning System." *Annals of Allergy* 29 (1971): 154.

Welshons, W. V., K. A. Thayer, B. M. Judy, J. A. Taylor, E. M. Durran, and F. S. vom Saal. "Large Effects from Small Exposures. I. Mechanisms for Endocrine Disrupting Chemicals with Estrogenic Activity." *Environmental Health Perspectives* 111, no. 8 (2003): 994–1006.

White, Jack. "How the EPA Was Made to Clean Up Its Own Stain—Racism." *Time*, Feb. 23, 2001.

White, Luise. "Poisoned Food, Poisoned Uniforms, and Anthrax, or, How Guerillas Die in War." In "Landscapes of Exposure: Knowledge and Illness in Modern Environments," edited by Gregg Mitman, Michelle Murphy, and Christopher Sellers, special issue, *Osiris*, 220–34. Chicago: University of Chicago Press, 2004.

Whorton, Donald, et al. "Investigation and Work-Up of Tight Building Syndrome." *Journal of Occupational Medicine* 29, no. 2 (1987): 142–47.

Whyte, William. *The Organization Man.* New York: Simon and Schuster, 1956.

Wiener, Norbert. *Use of Human Beings: Cybernetics and Society.* New York: Avon, 1967.

Wilson, Cynthia. *Chemical Exposure and Human Health.* Jefferson, N.C.: MacFarland, 1993.

——. "Disposable Cogs in a Disposable World." *Our Toxic Times*, Jan. 1996, 1–4.

Wilson, John. "Gots Misrepresents Workshop Conclusions on Internet." *Our Toxic Times*, May 1996, 1–6.

Winant, Howard. "White Racial Projects." In *The Making and Unmaking of Whiteness*, edited by Brigit Brander Rasmussen, Erick Klinenberg, Irene Nexica, and Matt Wray, 97–112. Durham, N.C.: Duke University Press, 2001.

Witteberg, Janice Strubbe. *The Rebellious Body: Reclaiming Your Life from Environmental Illness or Chronic Fatigue Syndrome.* New York: Plenum, 1996.

Working Women. *Warning: Health Hazards in the Office.* Cleveland: Working Women, 1981.

——, ed. *Race against Time: Automation of the Office.* Cleveland: National Association of Office Workers, 1980.

World Health Organization. *Indoor Air Pollutants: Exposure and Health Effects*. EURO Reports and Studies no. 78. Copenhagan: WHO Regional Office for Europe, 1982.

Wright, Gwendolyn. *Building the Dream: A Social History of Housing in America*. New York: Pantheon, 1981.

Yaglou, C. P., E. C. Riley, and D. I. Coggins. "Ventilation Requirements." *ASHVE Transactions* 42 (1936): 133–62.

Yates, JoAnne. *Control through Communication: The Rise of System in American Management*. Baltimore: Johns Hopkins University Press, 1989.

Zeff, Robbin Lee, Marsha Love, and Karen Stults, eds. *Empowering Ourselves: Women and Toxics Organizing*. Falls Church, Va.: Center for Health, Environment, and Justice, 1989.

Zenz, Carl. *Occupational Medicine: Principles and Practical Applications*. New York: Year Book Medical Publishers, 1988.

Zhu, Kangmin. "Letter to the Editor, 'Sick Building Syndrome': An Inappropriate Term." *Journal of Occupational Medicine* 35, no. 8 (1993): 752.

Zuboff, Shoshana. *The Age of the Smart Machine: The Future of Work and Power*. New York: Basic Books, 1988.

Zwillinger, Rhonda. *The Dispossessed: Living with Multiple Chemical Sensitivities*. Paulden, Ariz.: Dispossessed Project, 1998.

African Americans: environmental racism and, 118, 128–29; geographic distributions of privilege and, 114–15; job discrimination against, 39, 46, 55, 114, 127–29; "Negro Problem" and, 97, 98 (fig. 8), 100; in polluted communities, 105–6; surveys of, 97; urban development and, 114

AIDS activism, 156

Air conditioning, 2, 20–21, 33, 34, 141, 185nn.4–5

Air quality, 22, 82, 146–47, 185n.13, 193n.43, 203n.41

Althusser, Louis, 190n.2

American Academy of Environmental Medicine, 160, 162

American Conference of Government Industrial Hygienists (ACGIH), 88, 90

American Society of Refrigeration Engineers. See ASHRAE (American Society of Heating, Refrigerating, and Air-Conditioning Engineers); ASHVE (American Society for Heating and Ventilation Engineers)

Americans with Disabilities Act, 164

Anderson, Ann, 96

Anderson Laboratories, 121, 200n.39, 201n.41

Architecture: building functions vs. bodily functions in, 138; corporate prestige and, 30–31, 187n.33;

HVAC systems and, 32–33; International Style of, 30, 186n.27; machine aesthetic in, 30, 186n.28; Skidmore, Owings and Merrill (SOM) and, 30, 44, 187n.30; windows in, 22, 30, 32, 123. See also Office buildings; Sick building syndrome (SBS)

ASHRAE (American Society of Heating, Refrigerating, and Air-Conditioning Engineers), 29 (fig. 3), 32, 203n.41

ASHVE (American Society for Heating and Ventilation Engineers), 20–21, 23–24, 25–27, 88, 185nn.4–5

Assemblages: bodies in, 14, 58; buildings in, 13–14, 57, 58; chemical exposures as, 13; of comfort, 23–24, 26, 28, 32; definition of, 12, 183n.17; effects of chemicals on bodies, 88–91; of environmental comfort, 32; in experiment design, 24–25; historical regularities and, 13, 183n.19; of industrial hygiene, 87–88; of knowledge production, 23–24; male research subjects in, 26; material culture of office work and, 37, 79–80; materializations in, 7, 13–17, 57–58, 157–58, 175, 177, 181n.4; of popular epidemiology, 96; in toxicology, 91–92

Aub, Joseph, 87

Banham, Reyner, 185n.1
Bauer, Raymond, 136–37
Bauhaus, 30, 186n.27, 187n.29
Bay, Mia, 97
Becker, Franklin, 136–37
Bertoia, Harry, 43
Bodies: as assemblages, 14; build-
    ings and, 11, 19, 30, 159, 169, 174;
    communication system in, 173–
    74; as machines, 24–25; material-
    ization of, 17; MCS coping regimes
    and, 172–76; micromanagement
    of, 159, 170–71, 174; as multi-
    plicities, 11–12, 183n.14; odor
    removal from, 26–27, 179; office
    buildings compared to, 138; per-
    sonalized ecology, 161; standard-
    ization of, 25–27; stress-induced
    diseases and, 71, 75–78, 93,
    193n.43
Booth, Charles, 97
Boxer, Peter, 93
Braverman, Harry, 35
Brown, Phil, 96
Building Council on Indoor Air, 148
Building ecologists, 142–43, 146–
    48, 204n.47, 205n.55
Building Owners and Managers
    Association (BOMA), 144
Buildings systems approach, 146–
    48, 204n.47, 205n.55
Butler, Judith, 181n.4, 190n.2

Cannon, Walter, 87
Carbon monoxide experiments, 88,
    89 (fig. 6)
Carpeting, 49, 81, 121, 123–24, 125,
    200n.39
Carrier, Wallis, 20, 185n.4
Carson, Rachel, 102
Cassedy, Ellen, 60, 69
Center for Health, Environment and
    Justice. See Citizens Clearing-
    house for Hazardous Waste

Center for Indoor Air Research
    (CIAR), 82, 146
Chemical exposures: as assem-
    blages, 13; carcinogens and, 67,
    69, 106; from carpeting, 49, 81,
    121, 123–24, 125, 200n.39; com-
    pensation for, 58–59, 67, 91–92,
    126, 152, 164, 190n.6, 209n.41;
    consumerism and, 165; expert
    witnesses on, 161–62; govern-
    ment agencies and, 20, 28, 70–
    75, 82–83, 92, 95, 107, 116–17,
    138, 196n.34; historical ontology
    of, 7–8, 182nn.5–6; indoor pollu-
    tion and, 4–5, 125; legal action
    against, 126, 202n.53, 209n.41; as
    mass psychogenic illness (MPI),
    92–95, 126, 202n.53; materializa-
    tion of, 7, 181n.4; monitoring of,
    170–80, 212n.2; obstruction of
    analysis of, 117–18, 120–22, 127–
    30; threshold limit values (TLV)
    of, 88, 90–91, 92; uncertainty of,
    6–7, 9–10, 15, 58, 67–71, 83, 88–
    92, 124–27, 148–50; at Waterside
    Mall (EPA headquarters), 123–24.
    See also EPA; Privilege; Race;
    Toxicology
Circuit diagrams, 133–36, 135 (fig.
    20)
Citizens Clearinghouse for Haz-
    ardous Waste, 103, 106
Civil Rights Acts (1963, 1964), 55,
    115, 128
Clark, Adele, 181n.1
Clinical ecology, 159–62, 170
Coleman-Adebayo, Margaret, 128
Colligan, Michael, 93
Committee of Poisoned Employees
    (COPE), 124
Computer systems, 33, 51, 54, 56,
    66, 67, 68 (fig. 2), 193n.43
Congressional hearings: on chemi-

cal exposures, 124, 125, 127, 201n.40; Indoor Air Quality Act and, 144; on indoor pollution, 125, 127; on racial discrimination at EPA, 128

Consciousness raising, 62–65, 71–72, 191n.27

Copeland, Douglas, 52

Corporate sponsorship: of anti-MCS lobby, 162; of EPA research, 120, 121, 128–29, 130; of sick building syndrome (SBS) promotion, 147–48, 205n.55

Cowan, Ruth Schwartz, 181n.1

Cullen, Mark, 206n.1

Custodial workers, 52, 61, 208n.30

Cybercorp (James Martin), 135–36

Cybernetics, 16, 133–37, 141

Cyclex (tranquilizer), 93, 94 (fig. 7)

Daston, Lorraine, 182n.5

Daubert v. Merrill, 162, 201n.41

Deleuze, Gilles, 184nn.14, 16, 17, 185n.22, 208nn.21, 28, 211n.69

DeLillo, Don, 111, 122, 127, 201n.45

Donnay, Albert, 211n.744

Drinker, Cecil, 87, 88

Drinker, Philip, 20, 88

Drucker, Peter, 136

Du Bois, W. E. B., 97, 98 (fig. 8), 100, 106

DuPont Corporation, 49–50, 81

Eames, Charles and Ray, 43

Ecology: circuit diagrams of, 133–36, 135 (fig. 20); cybernetics and, 16, 133–37, 141; immune systems and, 124, 139, 160, 169–70, 171, 210n.59; information system as, 136; of natural systems, 139–40 (fig. 21); of organizations, 134, 136, 137; safe spaces and, 163–68, 174–76, 211n.74; of systems, 132–34, 160–61

Employee activism: American Federation of Government Employees (AFGE), 124; Committee of Poisoned Employees (COPE), 124; EPA Victims Against Racial Discrimination (EPAVRD), 128–29, 130. See also Local 2050 (National Federation of Federal Employees [NFFE]); 9to5 (National Organization of Women Office Workers)

Environmental chamber, 20, 21 (fig. 1), 23, 24–25

Environmental engineering: control in, 28; Defense Department funding of, 28; for information technologies, 33; odor removal and, 26–27, 179

Environmental illness, diagnosis of, 151–52, 206nn.1–2

Environmental Sensitivities Research Group (ESRI), 162, 209n.35

EPA: African Americans and, 115, 118, 128–29; building assessment approach of, to indoor pollution, 147; employee protests at, 124; environmental racism at, 128, 129; EPA Victims Against Racial Discrimination (EPAVRD) and, 128–29; Indoor Air Division of, 125, 147; indoor-pollution research at, 82; minority employment at, 115, 127; obstruction of research in, 117–18, 120–22, 127–30; popular epidemiology and, 107; research environment of, 116; sick building syndrome (SBS) defined by, 108. See also Local 2050 (National Federation of Federal Employees [NFFE])

EPA scientists: Committee of Poisoned Employees (COPE) and, 124; environmental activism of,

EPA scientists (*continued*)
125–27, 202n.53; interference with research of, 117–18, 120–22, 127–30; objectivity of, 119–20; production of uncertainty and, 120–21; reputation of, 116–17. *See also* Local 2050 (National Federation of Federal Employees [NFFE])

EPA Victims Against Racial Discrimination (EPAVRD), 128–29

Equal Rights Amendment, 85

Experiment design: assemblages in, 24–25; human physiology and, 24–25; imperceptibility and, 21–22, 100; regimes of perceptibility and, 10, 16, 24–25; sensory assessment and, 26–27; subject selection and, 24–25

Fairhill, Thomas, 90–91

Feminism: consciousness raising of, 62–65, 71–72, 191n.27; feminist science and, 181n.1; gendered divisions of labor and, 4; labor organizing and, 60–61, 191nn.10–11; on the new office technologies, 66; occupational health resources and, 66–67; professionalization of, 72, 193n.41; victim status and, 208n.30; working-class women and, 102–3

Feminization: of office work, 188n.4

Feral Robotic Dogs project, 212n.2

Foucault, Michel, 158–59, 181n.4, 182n.5, 183nn.17, 19, 184nn.14, 20, 187n.3, 191n.27, 208n.28

Framingham Heart Study, 75

Freeman, John, 134

Garrison, Barbara, 46

Gender: body/building nexus and, 159; building environments and, 5–6; chemical exposure and, 4, 208n.30; divisions of labor by, 4; domestic space and, 164, 173; employment discrimination by, 128; industrial hygiene and, 85; management and, 38, 40 (fig. 5), 55; mass psychogenic illness (MPI) and, 92–95, 126, 202n.53; MCS coping regimes and, 172–73; office building segregation by, 11; of office workers, 36, 187n.1; politics of activism and, 103; psychosomatic illness and, 152; of research subjects, 20, 25–26; spaces and, 159; stress-induced diseases and, 71, 75–78, 93, 193n.43; suburban corporate environment and, 31

Germ theory, 5, 22, 185n.13

Gibbs, Lois, 96, 103, 104 (fig. 19), 106, 116

Gorsuch, Ann, 117

Gots, Ronald, 162, 211n.74

Gropius, Walter, 30

Grossman, Rachel, 51–52

Guattari, Félix, 184nn.14, 16, 17, 185n.22, 211n.69

Gulf War syndrome, 145, 156–57, 167, 181n.3

Hacking, Ian, 182n.5

Haeckel, Ernst, 132

Hamilton, Alice, 72, 85–86, 87, 99, 195n.12

Hannan, Michael, 134

Haraway, Donna, 119–20, 208n.25

Harvard University, 20–21 (fig. 1), 54, 86, 87, 88, 136

Hasenyager, Bruce, 136

Hawthorne Experiments (Western Electric), 54, 186n.18

HBI (Healthy Buildings International), 146–48, 204n.47, 205n.55

Henderson, Lawrence J., 87

Hepler, Allison, 85, 194n.7

Herman Miller (office-furniture manufacturer), 43, 44, 47, 50
Historical ontology, 7–8, 10, 182nn.5–6
Historicity of experience, 57–80, 207n.17
Hitchcock, Henry Russel, 186n.27
Hull House, 72, 85, 86, 99, 100
Hutchinson, G. Evelynn, 133
Hysteria, 6, 7, 75, 126, 152

IBM (International Business Machine), 38, 47
Immune group (Internet) and Immuners, 167–68, 172, 174, 211n.65
Immune systems, 124, 139, 160, 169–70, 171, 210n.59
Imperceptibility: carpeting and, 49, 81, 121, 123–24, 125, 200n.39; of climate, 31–32; experiment design and, 21–22, 100; in knowledge production, 9–10, 182n.12; of low-level chemical exposures, 126–27; popular epidemiology and, 107; racialization of, 17; of Waterside Mall indoor pollution, 124, 125–26
Industrial hygiene: carbon monoxide experiments and, 88, 89 (fig. 16); chemical analyses and, 87–88; experimental physiology and, 87–88; occupational health investigators and, 141–42; in the Progressive Era, 86; safety standards for industrial chemicals and, 88; trustworthiness of female subjects and, 93–95; university laboratories for, 86–88, 90, 142; ventilation research and, 88
Instruction manuals, 37, 39 (fig. 4), 40 (fig. 5), 41, 42 (fig. 6)
International Program on Chemical Safety (IPCS), 211n.74
Internet, 167–68, 172, 174, 211n.65

Jencks, Charles, 187n.38
Jeremijenko, Natalie, 212n.2
Johnson, Philip, 186n.27

Kelley, Florence, 99, 100
Knoll, Florence, 43
Krauss, Celene, 116

Land, Edwin, 50
Latour, Bruno, 182n.5
Le Corbusier, 30, 186n.28
Leffingwell, William, 39 (fig. 4), 40 (fig. 5), 41, 42 (fig. 6)
Legionnaires' Disease, 138
Levin, Hal, 142
Lipsitz, George, 114
Local 2050 (National Federation of Federal Employees [NFFE]), 119–21; Committee of Poisoned Employees (COPE) and, 124; on corporate influence, 121–22, 127, 128–29, 130; environmental conditions in EPA building and, 122, 124, 201n.48; EPA scientists' environmental activism and, 124–27; public protests of, 124–25; support of, for EPA workers, 126; on tobacco smoke as health hazard, 205n.56
Love Canal, 66, 96, 104 (fig. 19), 105, 116

Male managers: college education of, 38; corporate prestige of, 30–31, 44–45 (fig. , 51, 187n.33; disbelief of, of office health hazards, 69, 70 (fig. 14); of ecosystems/ continual shakedown, 134; facilities management and, 139–40; instruction manuals for, 39 (fig. 4), 40 (fig. 5), 41, 42 (fig. 6); microtactics of, 64; of office interiors and, 136; organization of, 44, 45 (fig. 7), 51, 189n.29; patriarchalism of, 45–46, 65; scientific

Male managers (*continued*)
    management and, 38, 40 (fig. 5),
    54–55; women's relations with,
    39–41, 45–46, 65
Martin, Emily, 210n.59
Martin, James, 135–36
Mass psychogenic illness (MPI),
    92–95, 126, 202n.53
Massumi, Brian, 184nn.14–16
Materializations, 7, 13–17, 57–58,
    79–80, 157–58, 175, 177, 181n.4
Mayer, Hannes, 30
Mayo, Elton, 54
MCS (multiple chemical sensitivi-
    ties), 17–18; allergies and, 160;
    alternative healthcare and, 155,
    170–71; biochemical individuality
    and, 163; body/environment reac-
    tions and, 158–59; coping re-
    gimes and, 18, 172–76; diagnosis
    of, 152–53, 162–63, 206nn.1, 2, 4,
    207n.6; disability benefits for suf-
    ferers and, 209n.41; health insur-
    ance claims and, 152; as ideo-
    pathic environmental intolerance
    (IEI), 211n.74; as psychosomatic
    illness, 152, 172, 211n.65; as real
    disease, 152–54, 206n.4,
    207nn.6, 17; safe spaces for, 163–
    66; social abjection and, 152–54,
    157–58, 162, 177, 207n.17,
    211n.74; spiritual cause of, 171–
    72; symptoms as information,
    173–76; technologies of the self
    and, 158, 159, 174–75, 208n.28,
    211n.74; treatment centers for,
    162; women and, 152, 155, 157,
    162, 165, 172–73, 211n.65
MCS (multiple chemical sensitiv-
    ities) movement: cell metaphor
    for, 155; criticism of, 162, 211n.74;
    elsewhere within here, 157–58,
    208n.25; identity politics of, 155–

57; Immune group (Internet) and
    Immuners and, 167–68, 172, 174,
    211n.65; race and, 208n.30
MCSers (people with multiple chem-
    ical sensitivities): alternative med-
    icine and, 155, 170–71; bodies/
    building environment and, 169,
    174; body messages and self-
    diagnosis of, 174–76, 211n.74;
    Christian cells for, 16, 166, 171–
    72; cleaning products and, 164;
    consumerism of, 165; detoxifica-
    tion systems, 170; disability bene-
    fits, 209n.41; Ronald Gots and,
    162, 211n.74 ; immune systems,
    169, 210n.59; mental illness of,
    172, 211n.65; microbial inner-
    space, 170; safe spaces for, 163–
    66; spiritual cause of MCS, 171–
    72; stereotyping of, 210n.46;
    workplace accommodations for,
    209n.41, 210n.46
Mead, Margaret, 50
Media coverage: of chemical
    exposures, 124, 201n.49; of
    occupational illness, 73–74; sick
    building syndrome (SBS) in, 148
Medical community: alternative
    healthcare and, 155, 170–71; clini-
    cal ecology and, 161–62; diag-
    nosis of MCS (multiple chemical
    sensitivities) and, 152–53,
    206nn.1, 2, 4, 207n.6; on Gulf
    War syndrome, 145, 156–57, 167,
    181n.3; occupational medicine
    and, 90, 195n.8; standardization
    of physical examinations and,
    196n.17; on women's self-
    diagnoses, 70, 93–95, 211n.74
Mental illness. *See* MCS (multiple
    chemical sensitivities)
Middle class: air quality and, 22;
    anxieties of, 22, 26; chemical

exposure and, 208n.30; corporate management and, 31; gender divisions of work in, 45–46; migration of, to suburbia, 31; privilege of, 122–23; public health reform and, 22, 23; racial discrimination of, 39, 46, 55; on safe space, 165, 166–67; women in, 39, 40–41, 46, 55, 94, 166–67
Mills, C. Wright, 43
Montgomery Ward Headquarters, 49 (fig. 9)
Ms. magazine, 60
Multiplicities, 11–12, 133–34, 142, 148–50, 158–59, 184n.14

National Consumer League, 99
National Federation of Federal Employees (NFFE) Local 2050. *See* Local 2050 (National Federation of Federal Employees [NFFE])
National Medical Advisory Service, 162, 209n.36
National Organization of Women (NOW), 60
National Organization of Women Office Workers, 55, 60, 61
Nelson, George, 43, 44, 50
Newman, Penny, 105
Newtown Florists Club, 105
New York Radical Women, 63
9to5 (National Organization of Women Office Workers), 61, 63, 65, 67; Ellen Cassedy and, 60, 69; institutional character of, 72, 193n.41; movie on, 63, 191n.20; Karen Nussbaum and, 55, 60, 62, 69, 72, 75, 79, 193n.62; occupational health advocacy of, 67, 71; professionalization of, 72; stress defined by, 76–77 (fig. 15), 78; surveys and, 71–74. *See also* Project Health and Safety
NIOSH (National Institute of Occupa-

tional Safety and Health), 70–71, 74, 75, 82–83, 92, 95, 107, 196n.34
NO FEAR bill (Notification of Federal Employees Anti-discrimination and Retaliation Act), 129
Norton, Eleanor Holmes, 127–28
Nussbaum, Karen, 55, 60, 62, 69, 72, 75, 79, 193n.62

Occupational health investigators, 141–42
Occupational illness: compensation for, 58–59, 91–92, 190n.6; complaints of, 58; credibility of, 70–71; diagnoses of, 58–59, 70–71, 190n.6; publicity about, 73–74; stress-induced disease as, 76–78, 77 (fig. 15), 93, 193n.43; surveys of, 71–74, 193n.43
Odatus Immune System, 139
Odum brothers (Howard and Eugene), 133–34, 135 (fig. 20), 160–61
Office buildings: air conditioning in, 2, 20–21, 21, 33, 34, 141, 185nn.4–5; assemblages of, 13–14, 57; bodies compared to, 138; centralized environmental control and, 28, 30, 140–41; corporate prestige and, 30–31, 187n.33; custodial staff for, 52, 61, 131–32, 159, 208n.30; as efficient work spaces, 19; as empty shells, 32; facilities managers for, 139–40, 142; information technologies and, 33; interior design of, 43, 44, 45 (fig. 7); machine aesthetic and, 30; as multiplicities, 11, 183n.14; as natural spaces, 139–40 (fig. 21); private building investigators and, 142–43; privilege demarcated in, 11; smoking in, 31, 146–47, 187n.39, 204n.47, 205nn.55–56; in suburbia, 31; surveillance in, 41–42, 44, 45, 54–55, 140–41

Office furniture, 41–45, 47, 49
(fig. 9), 50, 137
Office interiors: accommodation for
MCSers and, 163; arrangements
of, 32, 35; bullpens and, 41–42;
carpeting in, 49, 81, 121, 123–24,
125, 200n.39; color schemes in,
49, 53; communication flow and,
47–50; cubicle systems in, 52–53,
54, 136; flexibility of, 32, 47, 48
(fig. 8), 50–51 (fig. 10), 137, 140–
41; furniture in, 41–45, 47, 49
(fig. 9), 50, 137; hierarchies in, 44,
45 (fig. 7), 51; layouts of, 32, 44–
49, 45 (fig. 7), 48 (fig. 8), 49
(fig. 9), 50 (fig. 10); open planning
of, 47–49, 48 (fig. 8), 50 (fig. 10),
52; participatory design in, 53–54;
segregation in, 11, 41–42, 115
Office Management (Leffingwell), 39
(fig. 4), 40 (fig. 5), 41, 42 (fig. 6)
Office work: compensation schedules for occupational illness and,
58–59, 91–92, 190n.6; definition
of sick building and, 144–45; efficiency of, 41, 42 (fig. 6); feminization of, 188n.4; information work
and, 33, 36, 43–44, 51, 61, 137; instruction manuals for, 37, 39 (fig.
4), 40 (fig. 5), 41, 42 (fig. 6); job
titles of, 38; machines and, 24–25,
36, 38, 39 (fig. 4), 40 (fig. 5), 41–
43, 42 (fig. 6); material organization of, 16; questionnaires for,
143–44, 203n.41; routine of, 37;
seating arrangements for, 41;
stress-induced disease and, 71,
75–78, 93, 193n.43; surveillance
of, 41–42, 44, 45, 54–55; teams in,
137; thermostat access and, 30, 33,
34; toxic chemical exposure from,
67–69; VDT systems and, 51, 54,
66, 67, 68 (fig. 12), 75, 193n.43

Operation systems management, 43
Organizational ecology, 134, 136, 137
Outsourcing, 51–52

Paigen, Beverley, 104 (fig. 19)
Perceptibility: of assemblages in toxicology, 91–92; production of, 10;
of racism, 112; regimes of, 10, 24–
25; surveys and, 71–74, 193n.43;
of threshold limit values (TLV),
92; of white noise, 111, 125–26,
127, 201n.45
Pittsburgh Survey 1906–7, 100
Popular epidemiology: assemblages
of, 96; community environmental activism and, 96, 197n.45;
grassroots environmentalism of,
106–7; imperceptibility in, 107;
instruction manual for, 103, 106;
Love Canal and, 66, 96, 104 (fig.
19), 105, 116; mapping of bio-
hazards and, 104 (fig. 19), 107;
mothers' community awareness
and, 103–5; risk calculus of, 101–
2, 106; scientific expertise and,
102; toxicology and, 96; working-
class women and, 102–4 (fig. 19).
See also Surveys
Private building investigators: backgrounds of, 142; as building ecologists, 142–43; buildings systems
approach of, 146–49, 204n.47,
205n.55; diagnostic tools of, 143,
149; medical imagery of, 143; risk
assessment and, 145–46; tobacco
industry and, 146–48, 204n.47,
205n.55; university industrial
hygienists compared with, 142
Privilege: chemical exposure and,
208n.30; geographic distributions
of, 114, 123, 127–28; objectivity as,
119–20; odorlessness as, 26–27,
179; racialization of, 17, 112–13,
127–29; suburbanization and, 31,

114–15; unmarkedness as sign of, 26; of white males, 20, 25–26, 28–29; of whiteness, 31, 105, 112–13, 115, 120, 122, 123. *See also* Male managers; Race

Processed World, 53 (fig. 11), 76, 77 (fig. 15)

Project Health and Safety: institutional character of, 72, 193n.41; on nonspecificity of office occupational health, 72; occupational health advocacy and, 71; research of, on toxic exposures, 67–69; use of term "stress" by, 75–76; surveys by, 72–73, 74

Propst, Robert, 33, 47, 50–51

Pruitt-Igoe housing development, 187n.38

Psychopathic illness, 6, 7, 75

Psychosomatic illness, 5–6, 75–78, 92–94, 126, 152–54, 172, 194n.61, 202n.53, 207n.17, 211n.65

Public health, 22, 23, 86, 101, 107

Questionnaires: on indoor air pollution, 125–26, 203n.41; multiple-choice format of, 144; office workers' awareness of problems and, 143–44

Quickborner Team, 47, 48 (fig. 8), 50 (fig. 10)

Race: advertisements and, 39; Civil Rights Acts (1963, 1964) and, 55, 115, 128; desegregation and, 115, 122, 128; environmental racism and, 105–6, 118–19, 123, 128–30; industrial hygiene and, 85; of maintenance workers, 52, 159, 208n.30; management positions and, 55; medicalization and, 211n.65; natural laws and, 97; "Negro Problem" and, 97, 98 (fig.

18), 100; of office workers, 36, 187n.1; outsourced positions and, 51–52; racial discrimination in hiring practices, 39, 46, 55, 115, 128–29; racialization of MCS movement and, 211n.65; racialization of privilege and, 17, 112–13, 127–29; scientific objectivity and, 120; spatial boundaries of, 115; suburbanization and, 31, 114–15, 122; whiteness and, 20, 25–26, 28–29, 31, 112–13, 115, 123

Randolph, Theron, 160, 161

Rapp, Rayna, 181n.1

Rea, William, 162

Reagan administration, 3, 32

Repace, James, 205n.56

Research subjects, 20, 24–26, 93–95, 125, 185n.13, 203n.41

Research Technical Advisory Committee on Physiological Reactions, 20

Robertson, Gary, 146, 147–48, 204n.4, 206n.50

Rogers, Sherry, 170

Safe spaces: body-building in, 174–76, 211n.74; entrepreneurialism and, 165; of home, as ecosystem, 165; in housing, 165–66; individualized biochemistry and, 164–65; information sharing on, 167–68; Internet as, 167; marketing to, 165; for MCSers, 163–66; middle class and, 165, 166–67; technologies of, 165

Sarachild, Kathie, 63

Schnelle brothers (Eberhard and Wolfgang), 47

Science and scientific research: corporate influence in, 121–22, 127, 128–29, 130; obstruction of, 117–18, 120–22, 127–30; opposing viewpoints in, 129; race and, 112.

Science and scientific (*continued*)
See also Popular epidemiology;
Surveys
Scientific management, 38, 40
(fig. 5), 54–55
Sellers, Christopher, 87
Selye, Hans, 76
Settlement houses, 85, 86, 96–97,
99, 100
Sharpton, Al, Rev., 128
Sick building syndrome (sbs): air filtration systems and, 139; buildings systems approach and, 146–
49, 204n.47, 205n.55; definition
of, 2, 6, 78–79, 144–45, 148; first
use of term, 83; health complaints
and, 1–2, 3; immune systems of,
139; in the media, 148; microbial
infections and, 138–39; nonspecificity of, 108–9; occupational
health investigators and, 141–42;
questionnaire as diagnostic tool
of, 143; tobacco industry and, 31,
82–83, 146–48, 187n.39,
204n.47, 205nn.55–56; vermin
infestations and, 138–39; workers
as sensors in, 144–45, 203n.41.
See also Architecture; Chemical
exposures; EPA; Office buildings;
Private building investigators;
Ventilation engineering; Waterside Mall (EPA headquarters)
Skidmore, Owings and Merrill
(SOM), 30, 44, 187n.30
Smoking, 4, 31, 82–83, 146–48,
187n.39, 204n.47, 205nn.55–56
Social abjection, 152–54, 157–58,
177, 207n.17
Social survey movement, 17, 71–74,
96–97, 102–4 (fig. 19), 193n.43
Specificity: of chemical exposure
identification, 58, 67–71, 88–92;
of occupational disease identification, 58–59; of office hazards, 59,
66–67; of physiological reactions
to chemicals, 88–92, 96; of sick
building syndrome (sbs), 108–9;
of surveys as analytical tool, 72–
74. See also Uncertainty
Spivak, Gayatri, 184n.23
Standardization: in architecture, 30;
comfort zone chart and, 25, 26,
27, 88; corporate management
and, 31; in questionnaires, 144;
reliability and, 25–26; of research
subject selection, 24–25; of surveys, 44
Stellman, Jeanne, 66–67, 76,
192n.31
Stress Test, The (Project Health and
Safety), 75–76
Surveys: of African Americans, 97;
Alice Hamilton and, 72, 85–86,
87, 99, 195n.12; on EPA working
conditions, 125–26, 201n.46;
experiential knowledge and, 73,
99–100; perceptibility of, 71–74,
193n.43; in popular epidemiology,
103–5; questionnaires and, 125–
26, 143–44, 144, 201n.46,
203n.41; in settlement houses,
96–97, 99; on sick building syndrome (sbs), 149; social survey
movement and, 17, 71–74, 96–
97, 102–4 (fig. 19), 193n.43; standardization in, 44; statistical
methods in, 73–74, 101; use of, by
private building investigators, 143,
149; women office workers and,
71–73, 96, 106, 193n.43; working-
class women and, 102–4 (fig. 19)
Systems ecology, 132–34, 160–61

Taylorism (Fredrick Taylor), 16, 37,
38, 41, 54, 188n.4
Technologies of the self, 158, 159,
174–75, 208n.28, 211n.74

Tepperman, Jean, 68 (fig. 12), 191n.11

Terr, Abba, 162, 202n.53

Threshold limit values (TLV), 88, 90–91, 92

Tobacco industry, 4, 31, 82–83, 146–48, 187n.39, 204n.47, 49, 205nn.55–56

Total Exposure Assessment Methodologies studies, 180

Toxicology: animals used in experiments on, 88, 90; assemblages in, 88–92; cancer and, 67, 69, 106; carpeting and, 49, 81, 121, 123–24, 125, 200n.39; chemical analyses and, 87; clinical ecology and, 159–62, 160, 161, 170; diagnostic tests and, 91–92; dose-response curve and, 88, 90, 180; experimental physiology techniques and, 87–88; imperceptibility and, 91; regulatory toxicology, 86; standards of proof in, 91; threshold limit values (TLV) and, 88, 90–91, 92

Toxic-waste activism, 17; environmental racism and, 118–19; Lois Gibbs and, 96, 103, 104 (fig. 19), 106, 116; Love Canal and, 66, 96, 104 (fig. 19), 105, 116; of women, 103, 105

Trinh Minh-Ha, 208n.25

Uncertainty: of chemical exposure identification, 6–7, 9–10, 15, 58, 67–71, 83, 88–92, 124–27, 148–50; of computers as occupational hazards, 66; mass psychogenic illness (MPI) and, 92–95, 126, 202n.53; obstruction of research as production of, 117–18, 120–22, 127–30; of occupational disease identification, 58–59; of stress identification, 71, 75–78, 93,

193n.43. *See also* MCS headings; Private building investigators; Surveys

Union Carbide Building, 44, 45 (fig. 7), 53, 137

Unionism, 60, 61, 112, 124, 148

Union WAGE, 60, 70 (fig. 14), 75

University industrial hygienists, 86–88, 90, 142

Van de Rohe, Mies, 30

Ventilation engineering: advertisements of, 29 (figs. 2, 3), 139–40 (fig. 21); air conditioning and, 2, 20–21, 33, 34, 141, 185nn.4–5; air quality and, 22, 82, 146–47, 185n.13, 193n.43, 203n.41; on buildings as natural systems, 139–40 (fig. 21); businesses and corporations and, 20; carbon dioxide and, 22, 185n.13; class anxiety and, 22; environmental chamber and, 20, 21 (fig. 1), 23, 24–25, 161, 162; government support for, 20; indoor climate fabricated by, 20; marketing of, 22, 23; research subjects and, 20, 24–26, 93–95, 125, 185n.13, 203n.41; white men and, 20, 28–29

Wallace, Lance, 125–26

Waterside Mall (EPA headquarters): carpeting of, 123–24, 125; environmental conditions in, 122; relocation of, 127; working conditions in, 123–24, 201n.46

White noise, 111, 125–26, 127, 201n.45

White Noise (DeLillo), 111, 122, 127, 201n.45

White women: chemical exposure of, 208n.30; health hazard evaluations of, 84; in MCS movement, 173, 211n.65; medicalization

White women (*continued*)
requests of, 173, 211n.65; as office
workers, 187n.1; personal safety
and, 166–67; in working class,
102–3
Whyte, William, 31, 187n.33
Wiener, Norbert, 47
Wilson, Cynthia, 207n.12
Winslow, C-E. A., 20
Women: chemical exposure of,
194n.7; chemical poisoning of,
192n.31; community awareness
of, 103–5; dress styles of, 40; hysteria and, 6, 7, 75, 126, 152; hysteria attributed to, 6, 7, 75; as
information workers, 51; labor
organizing of, 60; marriage and,
41; maternalism and, 85, 103–5;
MCS (multiple chemical sensitivities) and, 152, 155, 157, 162, 165,
172–73, 211n.65; middle-class
respectability and, 39, 40–41, 46,
55, 94, 166–67; in occupational
health, 72, 85–86, 87, 99,
195n.12; office furniture for, 41,
42 (fig. 6), 45; outsourced positions of, 51–52; popular epidemiology and, 102–4 (fig. 19);
promotions of, 41; psychosomatic
illness and, 5–6, 92–94, 152,
207n.17; sexual reproduction and,
66, 85; in toxic-waste activism,
96, 103, 104 (fig. 9), 105, 106, 116;
tranquilizers for, 93, 94 (fig. 17);
union representation of, at EPA,
124; as ventilation engineers,
185n.4; in women workers' movement, 55, 60, 62, 69, 72, 75, 79,
193n.62. *See also* Feminism;
Women office workers'
movement
Women office workers: African
Americans, 39, 46, 55; bullpen
arrangement for, 41–42; desir-
ability of office work, 38–39; dress
of, 40 (fig. 5); factory labor, 41, 42
(fig. 6), 55; feminization of office
work and, 38–41, 45–46, 55; as
girls, 38, 65; hierarchies of, 45–
46, 51–52; instruction manuals
for, 37, 39 (fig. 4), 40 (fig. 5), 41,
42 (fig. 6); machines operated by,
24–25, 38, 39 (fig. 4), 40 (fig. 5),
41–43, 42 (fig. 6); male managers
and, 39–41, 45–46, 65; mass psychogenic illness (MPI) and, 92–
95, 126, 202n.53; 9to5 (National
Organization of Women Office
Workers) and, 55; pink-collar class
of, 38–40, 210n.46; productivity
of, 54; racial discrimination in hiring practices and, 39, 46, 55, 128–
29; seating arrangements for, 41–
42, 45 (fig.7); segregation of, 41–
42; standardized motions and,
41–43; stress-induced diseases
and, 76–77 (fig. 15), 93, 193n.43;
surveys of, 71–73, 96, 193n.43;
unionism and, 60, 61, 112, 124;
wages of, 55. *See also* Feminism
Women Office Workers (WOW), 62–
63
Women office workers' movement:
consciousness raising and, 62–
65, 71–72, 191n.27; diversity lacking in, 61; emergence of, 60–61,
191nn.10, 11; on new office technologies, 66–67; popular epidemiology surveys and, 106; professionalization of, 72; rematerializations of office work by, 57–58.
See also 9to5 (National Organization of Women Office Workers)
Women's Occupational Health
Resource Center, 66–67
Working-class women: community

activism and empowerment of,
103–4 (fig. 19); as counterexperts,
102–4 (fig. 9); health clinics
established by, 102–3; organizations of, 105–6; scientific expertise of, 102–3; social surveys and,
102–4 (fig. 19)

*The Working Woman's Guide to Office
Survival* (9to5), 78
World Health Organization, 144–
45, 211n.74

Yaglou, Constantine, 20, 26, 88

Zuboff, Shoshana, 55

Michelle Murphy

is an assistant professor
in the History Department
and the Women and Gender
Studies Institute at the University
of Toronto.

*Library of Congress Cataloging-in-
Publication Data*

Murphy, Michelle (Claudette Michelle)
Sick building syndrome and the problem of
uncertainty : environmental politics, tech-
noscience, and women workers / Michelle
Murphy.
p. cm.
Includes bibliographical references and
index.
ISBN 0-8223-3659-6 (cloth : alk. paper)
ISBN 0-8223-3671-5 (pbk. : alk. paper)
1. Sick builidng syndrome—United States—
History. 2. Indoor air pollution—Health
aspects. 3. Buildings—Health aspects.
I. Title. [DNLM: 1. Sick Building Syndrome—
History—United States. 2. Air
Pollution, Indoor—United States.
WA 11 AA1 M 978s 2006]
RA577.5.M 87 2006
613′.5—dc22
2005027140